To MONA,

I believe that you wi
class professional in our fi

Fondly
yehuda

Handbook of Holistic Neuropsychological Rehabilitation

Handbook of Holistic Neuropsychological Rehabilitation

OUTPATIENT REHABILITATION OF TRAUMATIC BRAIN INJURY

Yehuda Ben-Yishay • Leonard Diller

OXFORD

UNIVERSITY PRESS

OXFORD
UNIVERSITY PRESS

Oxford University Press, Inc., publishes works that further
Oxford University's objective of excellence
in research, scholarship, and education.

Oxford   New York
Auckland   Cape Town   Dar es Salaam   Hong Kong   Karachi
Kuala Lumpur   Madrid   Melbourne   Mexico City   Nairobi
New Delhi   Shanghai   Taipei   Toronto

With offices in
Argentina   Austria   Brazil   Chile   Czech Republic   France   Greece
Guatemala   Hungary   Italy   Japan   Poland   Portugal   Singapore
South Korea   Switzerland   Thailand   Turkey   Ukraine   Vietnam

Published by Oxford University Press, Inc.
198 Madison Avenue, New York, New York 10016

www.oup.com

Library of Congress Cataloging-in-Publication Data
CIP data on file
ISBN 978-0-19-534125-6

9 8 7 6 5 4 3 2 1

Printed in USA
on acid-free paper

This book is dedicated to the memory of Herb Schreiber and to (the very much alive) CeCe, Karen, and Marnie Schreiber for their steadfast support—over the years—of the NYU-Rusk Day treatment program.

Acknowledgments

We wish to express our heartfelt thanks to our many patients for giving us permission to use videotaped excerpts from their personal "sessions" to help make this book a valuable teaching instrument. Likewise, we gratefully acknowledge the generous and able contributions of our colleagues Ellen Daniels-Zide, David Biderman, and Andrea Reyes (as well as others too numerous to be mentioned by name). We are especially indebted to Magnolia Davila for her ability to read hard-to-"decipher" handwritten pages and rendering them into neatly typed texts. Last but not least, our special thanks go to Joan Bossert, Editorial Director at the Oxford University Press, and to Tracy O'Hara, Development Editor. Their tireless efforts, patience, and outstanding editorial "touches" have helped make this a readable book.

Yehuda Ben-Yishay
Leonard Diller
New York, May 16, 2010

Contents

Introduction

This book is the culmination of three decades of intensive experience in holistic neuropsychological rehabilitation of young adults with traumatic brain injuries. Our aim in this book is not to provide a scholarly review of the state of the art. Nor is it to offer abstract theoretical formulations, or to critique current approaches by others to the remediation of deficits and the functional rehabilitation of people who sustained brain injuries. With few exceptions (such as Prigatano's *Principles of Neuropsychological Rehabilitation*) the focus of much of the literature in the field has been on providing evidence for the clinical efficacy of specific treatments. Our aim in this book is to articulate the rationale for, and to illustrate by means of videotaped excerpts, which are provided on the DVDs that accompany this book, the organizational as well as the programmatic aspects of the holistic approach to the neuropsychological rehabilitation of brain-injured individuals in the setting of a "therapeutic community."

By identifying our approach as "holistic," we mean precisely what Kurt Goldstein had in mind when he described his organismic theoretical formulations about the nature and the effects of brain injury, and the rehabilitation endeavor. The central thesis of the holistic approach is this: To restore a brain-injured individual to function optimally, it is necessary to establish a therapeutic milieu that is experienced by the injured person as "safe" (in the sense that, the chances for the occurrence of "catastrophic" responses by the patient to perceived threats will be reduced). In this "safe" environment, the injured individual can, gradually, begin to use still intact capacities and learn, optimally, compensatory skills. The compensation process, thus, helps the person to attain an enhanced functional adjustment. Improvements in their functional adjustment will facilitate those individuals' calm acceptance of the life-altering changes, or limitations, that were caused by their brain injury. Acceptance—it is hoped—will also help these individuals to find new meaning in their lives after rehabilitation.

We readily concede that NYU-Rusk Institute day program could scarcely be described as the "typical" program since the number of patients in any given 20-week treatment cycle rarely exceeds 12 persons who have been carefully selected, and each of our patients receives an average of 1,000 hours of treatment, before actually commencing his or her work or academic trials. One may, therefore, legitimately ask whether or not the overall philosophy of our program, indeed even some of the remedial and therapeutic techniques that are employed in our setting, could be incorporated in other (more conventional types of) programs. Based on our experience, over more than three decades, we are convinced that despite the differences between our program and other programs, much could be shared with colleagues in the field. This conviction has been reinforced by the fruitful exchanges that have taken place, since the inception of our program, in hundreds of intensive workshops, or in visits to our program by working clinicians from different countries. Certainly, some questions concerning the applicability of the philosophy, as well as some of the remedial and therapeutic techniques as they are practiced in our program, remain to be systematically examined in the future.

We believe that the different programmatic, remedial, and therapeutic aspects of our program, as they are described in this text and illustrated by judiciously edited videotaped excerpts, will be found useful by different professionals in the field of rehabilitation. For the administrator, who may wish to establish a holistic program—aimed at supplementing already existing services for brain-injured patients—this book provides concrete information concerning the nature, scope, the cost, as well as the levels of staff expertise that will be required to establish a holistic program of this kind. For the academic instructor, whose task is to educate future professionals in the field, this volume can serve as a useful reference book. For the clinical service evaluator, this volume provides significant clues as to what to look for in order to determine whether or not a particular program under review responds adequately to the special needs of brain-injured people in rehabilitation.

We do not claim that ours is the only useful approach to the rehabilitation of brain-injured individuals. Nor do we feel that the holistic approach is suited for all brain-injured people. We wish, however, to point out several merits of the model. First, our approach has withstood the test of time. Second, our program has produced successful outcomes in hundreds of cases since 1978. Third, with some modifications—to accommodate different "local" needs or different cultural settings—our approach has been successfully applied in the United States as well as in other countries.

We have opted deliberately to communicate our thoughts in an informal, "conversational" style in this book. Our aim is to provide working clinicians with an experience of "you are there." Our aim is also to render this book easily "readable" by people who are not used to reading journal articles or scholarly texts. We readily admit, however, that a book, even when it is accompanied by illustrative video clips, is but a poor substitute for either attending an intensive workshop or—better yet—to visiting and observing our program firsthand.

In deciding which of our patients to select in order to illustrate various clinical issues, we have deliberately chosen those individuals who made it possible to clearly show how temperamental factors, personality traits, and specific life experiences interacted with the patients' organic impairments, and their sequelae—in a way that produced the unique ways that the brain injuries of those individuals manifested themselves in their behavior. Furthermore, we freely admit that the chapter about the ultimately successful responses of several "problematic" patients to our program is intended to demonstrate that when one possesses the "right clinical tools," the "right therapeutic milieu," and the necessary time, it is possible to obtain successful outcomes, even in patients who, in more conventional settings, may fail to respond to rehabilitative interventions.

We, likewise, wish to emphasize that our clinical formulations, as well as the DVD illustrations, are not meant to be formulaic, or "prescriptive," in nature. Rather, they are offered merely as templates that practicing clinicians—who may wish to emulate them—ought to "translate" into their own personal style of clinical communication. In addition, the list of references at the end of chapters is highly selective. It includes some of our own publications or the publications of others that influenced our thinking about particular issues at hand.

Some readers may wish to receive evidence-based information about the efficacy of our general approach to the rehabilitation of mildly to moderately impaired individuals with a brain injury. We remind those readers that in their authoritative review, Cicerone and associates (see list of references following the first chapter) have pointed out that holistic approaches to cognitive rehabilitation are recommended not on the basis of controlled clinical trials, but on the basis of clinical consensus: controlled clinical trials are extremely difficult to conduct due to problems in acquiring well-matched groups of subjects. A more salient point, however, is that studies that test the efficacy of given remedial or therapeutic techniques rarely, if ever, provide sufficient guidance as to how to exactly apply techniques in specific program settings, and that the application of controlled studies to actual patient populations remains as yet an unsolved problem.

Finally, while admittedly much more work remains to be accomplished, we believe that by embodying Kurt Goldstein's conceptual ideas, systematically studying the efficacy as well as the effectiveness of (specially developed) remedial and psychotherapeutic techniques, and monitoring the application of these techniques in different programs (in the U.S. and other countries), the NYU holistic model helps to move the field of neuropsychological rehabilitation from what (essentially) was an empirically based clinical endeavor to (eventually) a rational theoretically based endeavor.

Chapter 1   *Evolution of Psychological Interventions in Rehabilitation*

Because cognitive (and overall neuropsychological) rehabilitation is a relatively new area of specialization (in the context of the field of medical rehabilitation), we may ask: How did the methods and ideas originate for managing the problems of living with limitations that are the consequences of acquired brain injury?

Ideas about how to help people to deal with difficulties they experience during the onset of head injuries go back to ancient times, but little is mentioned, in the ancient accounts, about the management of problems after the acute phase of the brain injury.

Modern approaches borrowed ideas from two sources: (1) clinical experience with different neurological syndromes; and (2) the public-health perspective and its interest in the treatment of people who suffered brain injuries, which over the years have influenced expectations concerning the types of services that should be provided under the "umbrella" of rehabilitation. Each of these is briefly discussed in the sections that follow.

Experience with Different Neurological Syndromes

Broca identified different patterns of language dysfluency (i.e., inability to speak or write smoothly or easily) in people with aphasia. He showed that a relationship exists between this type of problem and left-hemispheric brain impairment. Broca also suggested methods of "reeducation." The rich tradition of neurology in Germany and the fact that during World War I Germany suffered a very high rate of war casualties with head wounds produced two influential approaches. In the first major approach, Poppelreuter clarified the nature of visual perceptual difficulties and suggested ways of dealing with perceptual impairments. Poppelreuter was also interested in helping such war-injured veterans to return to work. The second major approach was developed by Kurt Goldstein. He focused on what we, today, consider to be failures that are specifically associated with impairments of frontal-lobe functioning. Goldstein's primary focus was on understanding the nature of behavioral and cognitive impairments following a brain injury, on the basis of extensive clinical observations of pathological behaviors that were manifested by head-injured war veterans.

Goldstein's place in the history of our field cannot be overemphasized for the following reasons:

1. Goldstein interpreted the many pathologic behaviors he observed in World War I head-injured veterans (such as the problems that resulted from extreme concreteness of thinking and its opposite—the inability to reason abstractly or symbolically) from the perspective of his "organismic" theoretical formulations about human nature. Accordingly, Goldstein argued that deficient behaviors ought to be seen as special cases of a failure to respond to environmental challenges in a normal way. In other words, Goldstein saw pathological phenomena as unsuccessful attempts to cope (he called this "coming to terms") following a brain injury, within the range of the capabilities and inherent tendencies of the normal human organism.

2. Goldstein's second major contribution to the development of the field of neuropsychological rehabilitation was his dramatic demonstration that, by altering the external visual and cognitive challenges of tasks that brain-injured people were initially unable to cope with (such as when facilitatory cues were provided), they now proved able to perform those tasks. This idea of Goldstein has been one of the central guiding principles of our own holistic, "therapeutic milieu" program many years later. (Since the existence of our program, more than 400 patients have "graduated.") Goldstein's idea also served as a forerunner of contemporary approaches to errorless learning. A holistic program advances the idea of errorless learning beyond psychometric types of tasks.

Like many great doctors of his day, Goldstein's attempts to help his patients resume work and better adapt to their family lives paved the way to our present-day conception of rehabilitation following brain injury. No wonder, therefore, that Luria (the renowned Russian psychologist of post–World War II fame) declared Goldstein to be the "father of modern neuropsychology."

At the beginning of the nineteenth century, Itard, who worked with children, helped to lay the groundwork for developing special education approaches to help children who were born with cognitive limitations. Itard's work inspired the development of the field of modern special education, which now is part of the practices of members of the teaching profession. By focusing on helping cognitively challenged (previously identified as mentally retarded) children to learn, to perform daily-life tasks, and to better adapt to family living, the field of special education devoted itself to helping individuals with limited abilities to compensate for their limitations. The concern of the special educators today also includes the education of the members of the family of the limited individual, and counseling them how to manage the child in the context of family living, as well as efforts to help such individuals to become productive. In other words, to help intellectually challenged people to compensate for their limitations in order to integrate socially within the limits of their capacity to adapt and to become integrated in society. Hence, the field of special education has much in common with the field of neuropsychological rehabilitation as it is practiced today.

The Influence of "Public-Health" Perspective on the Treatment of People with Acquired Brain Injury

The foundations of modern approaches to the rehabilitation of people with acquired brain injury grew out of the treatment of these injuries during and after World War I. Germany took the lead not only because of its many head-injured casualties and the advanced state of neurology in that country, but also because of the enlightened social policies that were introduced by Bismarck (the first chancellor of modern Germany) about three decades earlier. (Bismarck's ideas concerning the role of the state in providing healthcare benefits to its citizens extended beyond the stage of acute hospital care.)

While most of the European medical rehabilitation services were severely limited, as a result of the great social and economic dislocations that followed World War I, in the United States the major efforts in the area of brain injury were directed primarily toward conducting case studies capable of explaining the brain–behavior relationship. But, from the standpoint of the public health concern with developing and delivering medical and rehabilitative services to people with acquired brain injury, little or no progress was made between the two world wars in the United States.

World War II (and the war between Russia and Finland that preceded it) stimulated a revival of the interest in working with individuals with traumatic brain injuries. Luria's published ideas, based on his experiences with head-injured war veterans, had a profound effect on the thinking of clinical neuropsychologists everywhere.

And with the development of high-speed highway systems in the United States, there was an increase in motor vehicle accidents in the 1960s and 1970s, which led to increasing public concern.

This increased public concern with developing medical and neuropsychological services for head trauma victims was aided by reported findings from similar efforts with Israeli head-injured war veterans, following the 1973 "Yom Kippur" war. Goldstein's holistic ideas concerning the diagnosis and the treatment of persons with acquired brain injury were reintroduced, leading to further development in the United States as well as in other countries (e.g., Israel, South Africa, and Europe) of programs dedicated to the rehabilitation of brain-injured individuals.

From a "bird's-eye view," the development of our field can be seen as having had different phases, or stages. Thus, from 1970 to 1980 the main emphasis was on demonstrating that cognitive-remedial and vocational rehabilitative techniques are efficacious. From 1980 to 1990, the primary emphasis was on measuring the outcomes of neuropsychological rehabilitation in terms of the number of brain-injured people who returned to work; the types of work they proved able to engage in following rehabilitation; and objective measures of the quality of life and social reintegration they managed to achieve. And since the 1990s, there has been a major shift from examining the outcomes of intensive neuropsychological rehabilitation in terms of ("external") objective measures to the subjective experiences of the brain-injured people, during and with the rehabilitative process itself, and the individual's appraisal of the meaning of life after rehabilitation. This, then, brings us full circle; since, as Goldstein often declared, the aims of neuropsychological rehabilitation are not only to help brain-injured people to become able to better adapt in their daily lives, but also to help them find meaning in their lives after rehabilitation.

Suggested Readings

Benton, A. L. (1989). Historical notes on the post concussion syndrome. In H. S. Levin, H. M. Eisenberg, and A. L. Benton (Eds.), *Mild head injury*. New York: Oxford University Press.

Ben-Yishay, Y. (1986). Reflections on the evolution of the therapeutic milieu concept. *Neuropsychological Rehabilitation 6*, 327–342.

Ben-Yishay, Y. (2007). Selected early publications on the Holistic Day Program. New York: N.Y.U. Medical Center, Rusk Institute BIDTP, BBIRR Publication.

Ben-Yishay, Y., & Daniels-Zide, E. (2000). Examined lives: Outcomes after holistic rehabilitation. *Rehabilitation Psychology, 45*(2), 112–129.

Cicerone, K. D., & Wood, J. C. (1987). Planning disorder after closed head injury: A case study. Archives of Physical Medicine and Rehabilitation, 68, 11–115.

Goldstein, K. (1942). *After effects of brain injuries in war: Their evaluation and treatment*. New York: Grune and Stratton.

Goldstein, K. (1952). *Human nature in the light of psychopathology*. Cambridge, MA: Harvard University Press.

Goldstein, K. (1959). What we can learn from pathology for normal psychology? *Proceedings of conference sponsored by U.S. Dept of HEW*. June 13, 36–135.

Itard, J. M. G. (1962). *The wild boy of Averon* (G. Humphrey, Trans.). New York: Appleton Century Crofts.

Chapter 2 *Essentials of Holistic Neuropsychological Rehabilitation*

In this chapter, we discuss some of Kurt Goldstein's holistic views concerning the diagnosis and treatment of brain-injured individuals—as they have been interpreted, operationalized, and clinically applied by us in the setting of our therapeutic community-type of day program.

These ideas have been serving as the conceptual foundations of our program and have been guiding our clinical-rehabilitative work throughout the years. Reduced to basics and stated succinctly, they are as follows:

1. Before beginning the efforts to rehabilitate brain-injured people, it is necessary to identify (and to understand) the causes for their failure to function adequately following the brain injury.

As a first step, clinicians must identify the underlying causes for a person's failure to function, or to perform, as normally expected. As is shown by Figure 2.1, a failure to function adequately after a brain injury can be the result of one or a combination of three basic causes.

One of the major causes is an organic lesion, or the dysfunction, in a specific region of the person's brain. A second cause of a functional failure is the disuse by the injured individual of some of his or her still intact (i.e., unimpaired by the injury) abilities. This disuse is not a conscious phenomenon. Rather, it is the result of (what Goldstein called) an "organismic defense," which is an automatic response by the brain-injured person to prevent the occurrence of a "catastrophic" reaction. A "catastrophic" response is a complete breakdown in person's ability to cope, that is, to satisfactorily deal with some challenge in the environment. The disuse of still intact abilities, therefore, can be

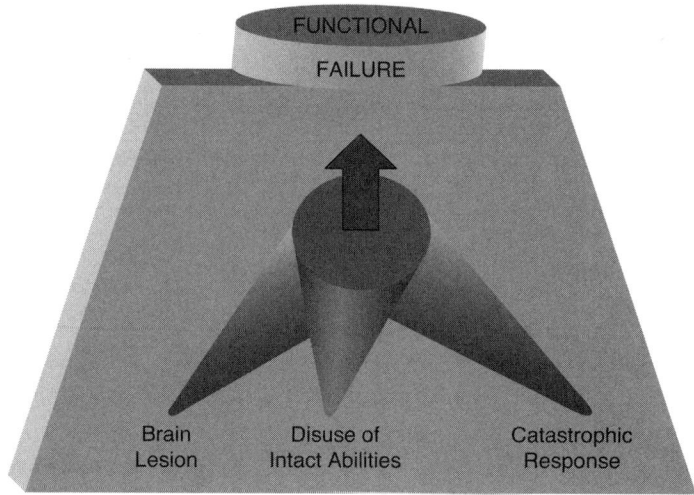

Figure 2.1.

Causes of functional failure

viewed as an organismic protective mechanism (which we humans share with other living organisms in the animal kingdom). We may also describe this as a "conservative" mechanism that is automatically activated when there exists a threat to the organism's existence (such as following severe injuries). The third cause of a failure to function is the organism's actually being in a "catastrophic" state.

But, while a "catastrophic response" is only the most extreme form of a failure to adequately cope with challenges, there are less extreme forms of insufficient coping abilities when individuals must face challenges in their daily lives. We can, thus, find three general ways of adjusting to, or coping with, different situations in life. (Goldstein called this "coming to terms with reality.") These coping styles can be described as ranging along a continuum, as shown in Figure 2.2.

At the successful end of coping with problem-solving situations, we find individuals who can assume a logical, deliberative (i.e., a calmly reasoning) mental attitude. A somewhat less efficient manner of approaching a problem-solving situation—still within the deliberative range—is the individual's engagement in a "trial-and-error" style of problem-solving activity. The next stage in the continuum can be described as the "transitional" stage. In the transitional stage, the individual may

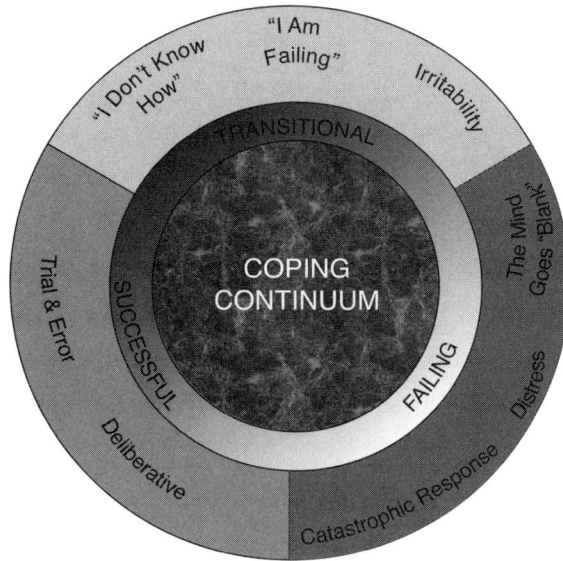

Figure 2.2.

The coping continuum

become aware of the fact that he or she does not know how to proceed toward solving the problem. But the individual remains still in control of his or her emotions (intending to keep trying). This may be followed by a disturbing thought ("I cannot do this!") and by perplexity, confusion, or irritability. Irritability, Goldstein taught us, in a brain-injured individual, is a warning signal that the person may soon enter the zone of a failure to cope. One version of a failure to cope is the experience of the mind going "blank." More disturbing variations of a failure to cope are distress, anxiety, or agitation, which are manifestations of a "catastrophic response."

The following two examples illustrate special forms of "catastrophic" responses. In the first case, a woman—the mother of a son at war—observed from her kitchen window, the local priest and an army officer approaching her porch. She stepped out, took the envelope that was handed to her by the officer, and promptly fainted. (The letter was a telegram informing her that her son died in battle.) The second situation involved an elderly college professor in biological sciences who suffered a stroke that paralyzed his left leg. The gentleman was engaged in an amiable conversation with a psychologist. The psychologist asked the old professor: "Why are you unable to stand and walk on your own?" "Because I am tired," answered the professor. The psychologist then proceeded: "Your doctor explained to me why your left leg is unable to hold you up." As soon as the psychologist mentioned the words "thrombosis" and "hemiplegia," the professor fell fast asleep. Minutes later, the gentleman woke up and the pleasant conversation between the two men continued as if nothing happened just minutes before.

2. In a functional failure, neurologic, cognitive, and personality factors always interact and influence one another. When we attempt to understand the meaning of a functional failure in an individual with brain injury, it is important to keep in mind that a neurologic impairment, leading to a functional failure, is always influenced—in an obvious, or subtle, manner—by the person's cognitive deficits that are associated with the brain injury; and both are influenced by that person's unique personality characteristics. This is illustrated by Figure 2.3.

Accordingly, when we diagnose in a brain-injured person disturbances in the sense of self (also known as "identity"), which are manifested as losses in the person's self-confidence, lowered self-esteem, or interferences in the person's ability to learn and to work, or problems in the area of interpersonal relationships, it is important to keep in mind that such

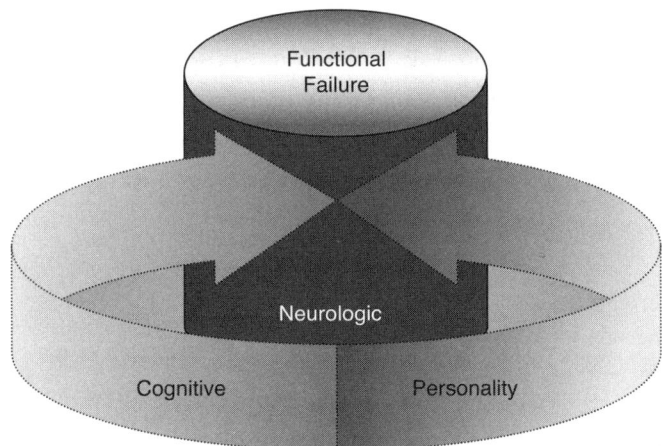

Figure 2.3.

Neurologic, cognitive, and personality factors determine the way a functional failure manifests itself

problems are always expressed in the person's functional life in unique ways. Figure 2.4 depicts these interactions.

Workers in the field must guard against committing errors in diagnosis that typically inexperienced clinicians are prone to commit. We must be vigilant not to arrive at misdiagnoses merely on the basis of the specific symptomatic manifestations or the failure to perform, or the inadequate performance of specific tasks by a brain-injured individual. We must ask what the more basic (underlying) causes of such symptoms are. We may illustrate this by looking at three brain-injured individuals, all of whom sustained frontal lobe injuries resulting in severe impulse control problems, and all of whom were evaluated by inexperienced neuropsychologists. The first of the three disinhibited patients performed block design tests hastily, carelessly, and in a defective manner. He was diagnosed (among other problems) as having a "constructional praxis" deficit. The second patient expressed himself, during a clinical interview, in ways that led the examiner to conclude that this person lacked "completely" "the ability to empathize with others." And the third patient produced a written statement that was full of incomplete sentences and grammatical and syntactic errors. Upon reading this statement the examiner diagnosed the patient as having "aphasic problems."

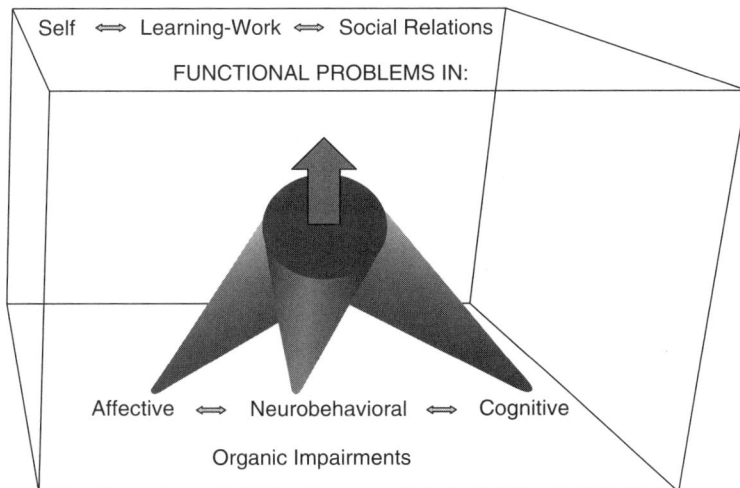

Figure 2.4.
Different combinations of organic impairments produce different types of functional deficits

Subsequently, all three patients received intensive remedial interventions aimed at helping them to compensate for their impulse control problem. When they were retested, the first patient performed the block design test normally. The second proved able to interact empathically with his peers and family members. The third (who was labeled initially "aphasic") was able to write and speak his mind normally.

The "lesson" learned from the preceding examples is obvious. Three inexperienced psychologists who observed correctly pathological symptomatic manifestations failed to notice the more basic impulse control problem of the patients they evaluated.

3. When attempting to rehabilitate brain-injured individuals, it is necessary to evaluate which of the brain-injured person's problems can be ameliorated, that is, improved, by remedial interventions and which (as Goldstein said) should be "left alone." An easy-to-understand example is when the patient's attention concentration deficits can be ameliorated by remedial training, but his or her slowed speed of performance (due to brain stem damage) should be "left alone," since the problem may never lend itself to ameliorative training.

4. It is also important to evaluate which of the existing psychotherapeutic approaches (and techniques) are suitable and which are not suitable for brain-injured individuals.

In view of the particular cognitive and emotional limitations that are typically produced by their brain injuries, insight-producing "talking therapies" are rarely effective in the case of brain-injured individuals, and alternative forms therapeutic interventions ought to be developed to help such individuals.

Implications for Diagnosis

■   The performance of a single task, or test, in a defective manner is not, in and of itself, proof of the presence of brain injury.

■   But, the opposite is also true: A normal performance of a single task, or test, does not rule out the possibility that in other areas of functioning the individual may be impaired by a brain injury.

■ Therefore, whether or not a person's functioning may be impaired (following a brain injury) in some way must be assessed by a variety of tests and in different situations. Accordingly, a comprehensive evaluation should consist of:

1. Structured and unstructured interviews with the patient, as well as his or her significant others, to ascertain whether the injury may have produced major alterations in the patient's functional competencies or "personality".

2. Observations of the patient's functioning in his or her "naturalistic" environment, as well as in unfamiliar surroundings.

3. Formal testing situations capable of sampling the integrity of the injured individual's basic neuropsychological functions and higher level cognitive functions; the ability to learn and retain new information; and the individual's interpersonal skills.

4. Evaluation of the person's ability to benefit from individualized or group remedial interventions designed to help him or her to compensate for deficits.

Implications for Treatment

To achieve optimal outcomes, remedial interventions should be focused simultaneously, in a coordinated and complementary way, on:

1. Helping the brain-injured person to compensate (as much as possible) for basic neuropsychological deficits, such as impulse-control problems or difficulties in initiating; difficulties in persisting at purposeful behaviors; and focusing and maintaining attention and concentration.

2. Helping the individual to compensate for difficulties in effectively processing information; memory problems; interferences with his or her higher level reasoning abilities; and addressing therapeutically problems with the person's emotional reactions to the consequences of the brain injury, or difficulties in the interpersonal sphere.

To achieve optimal results from neuropsychological rehabilitative efforts, it is necessary to organize the environment for the brain-injured individuals (and the training challenges) so that the chances of their experiencing failure in coping will be minimized. (This is discussed in some detail in Chapter 3.)

Suggested Readings

Barth, J. T., & Boll, T. J. (1981). Rehabilitation and treatment of central nervous system dysfunction: A behavioral medicine perspective. In C. K. Prokop & L. A. Bradley (Eds.) *Medical psychology* (pp. 242–259). New York: Academic Press.

Ben-Yishay, Y., Ben-Nachum, Z., Cohen, A., Gross, Y., Hoofien, D., Rattok, J., et al. (1977). Digest of a two-year comprehensive clinical research program for outpatient head injured Israeli veterans. *N.Y.U. Rehabilitation Monograph 64*, 128–176.

Ben-Yishay, Y., & Diller, L. (1983). Cognitive deficits. In M. Rosenthal, E. R. Griffith, M. R. Bond, & J. D. Miller (Eds.), *Rehabilitation of the head injured adult* (pp. 167–183). Philadelphia: F.A. Davis.

Ben-Yishay, Y., & Diller, L. (1983). Cognitive remediation. In M. Rosenthal, E. R. Griffith, M. R. Bond, & J. D. Miller (Eds.), *Rehabilitation of the head injured adult* (pp. 367–380). Philadelphia: F.A. Davis.

Ben-Yishay, Y. & Prigatano, G. P. (1990). Cognitive remediation. In M. Rosenthal, E. R. Griffith, M. R. Bond, & J. D. Miller (Eds.). *Rehabilitation of the adult and child with traumatic brain injury* (2nd ed., pp. 393–408). Philadelphia: FA Davis.

Ben-Yishay, Y., Rattok, J., Lakin, P., Piasetsky, E., Ross, B., Silver, S., et al. (1985). Neuropsychological rehabilitation: The quest for a holistic approach. *Seminars in Neurology, 5*, 252–259.

Boll, T. J., O'Leary, D. S., & Barth, J. T. (1981). A quantitative and qualitative approach to neuropsychological evaluation. In C. K. Prokop & L. A. Bradley (Eds.), *Medical Psychology* (pp. 68–79). New York: Academic Press.

Diller, L. (1985). Neuropsychological rehabilitation. In M. Meier, A. L. Benton, & L. Diller (Eds.) *Neuropsychological rehabilitation* (pp. 3–17). New York: Guilford.

Diller, L. (1994). Finding the right combinations: Changes in rehabilitation over the past five years. In A. L. Christensen and B. P. Uzzell (Eds.),

Brain injury and neuropsychological rehabilitation (pp. 1–16). Mahwah, NJ: Lawrence Erlbaum.

Diller, L., & Ben-Yishay, Y. (1988). Stroke and traumatic brain injury: Behavioral and psychosocial considerations. In J. Goodgold (Ed,), *Rehabilitation Medicine* (pp. 135–143). Washington, DC: CV Mosley.

Diller, L., & Gordon, W. (1981). Interventions for cognitive deficits in brain injured adults. *Journal of Consulting and Clinical Psychology, 49,* 822–833.

Goldstein, K. (1942). *After effects of brain injuries in war: Their evaluation and treatment.* New York: Grune and Stratton.

Goldstein, K. (1959). Notes on the development of my concepts. *Journal of Individual Psychology, 15*(1), 5–19.

Goldstein, K. (1959). What we can learn from pathology for normal psychology. In G. Leviton (Ed.), *Proceedings of conference sponsored by U.S. Dept. of HEW,* June 13, 36–135.

Hoffien, D., & Ben-Yishay, Y. (1982). Neuropsychological therapeutic community rehabilitation of severely brain injured adults. In E. Lahav (Ed.), *Psycho-social research in rehabilitation* (pp. 87–99). Tel-Aviv, Israel: Ministry of Defense, Department of Rehabilitation Publishing House.

Lezak, M. (2004). *Neuropsychological assessment* (4th ed.). New York: Oxford University Press.

Moore, M. S., & Mateer, C. A. (1989). *Introduction to cognitive rehabilitation.* New York: The Guilford Press.

Prigatano, G. P. (1999). *Principles of Neuropsychological Rehabilitation.* New York: Oxford University Press.

Prigatano, G. P., & Ben-Yishay, Y. (1999). Psychotherapy and psychotherapeutic interventions in brain injury rehabilitation. In M. Rosenthal, E. R. Griffith, J. S. Korntzer, & B. Pentland (Eds.). *Rehabilitation of the adult and child with traumatic brain injury,* (3rd ed.), 271–283. Philadelphia: F.A. Davis.

Chapter 3   *Elements of a Treatment Cycle*

This chapter (1) outlines the principal elements of a treatment cycle in the holistic day program; (2) points out the major benefits that are obtained when the remedial and therapeutic interventions are structured and organized in a therapeutic milieu; (3) demonstrates how the complementary cognitive-remedial, therapeutic, and "community" interventions—during a program day and throughout the entire cycle—help brain-injured individuals to gradually realize individualized clinical objectives; (4) explains how the compensatory process unfolds (i.e., takes place) in a cumulative spiral-like fashion; and (5) illustrates (by selected, edited videotaped samples) how the different program treatments are applied clinically.

General Elements

Optimal Time Frame. We have found that the optimal time frame for a treatment cycle is a 20-week time period. Within this time frame, effective remedial interventions—5 hours a day, 4 days a week, or a minimum of 400 hours of treatments per cycle—can take place. Progress can be evaluated in an ongoing way, to determine both the rate of each individual's progress as well as the qualitative (i.e., the clinical meaningfulness) of that progress.

The "Clinical Council." The professional staff acts as a "clinical council." As shown in Figure 3.1, the professional staff is one of the three principal "partners" in the "therapeutic community" type of program. In this setting, the staff operates as a "clinical council" that deliberates and jointly formulates both the overall clinical strategy as well as the specific "tactics" (i.e., procedures) that should be followed by all the staff members, under an explicitly formulated and agreed-upon master treatment plan.

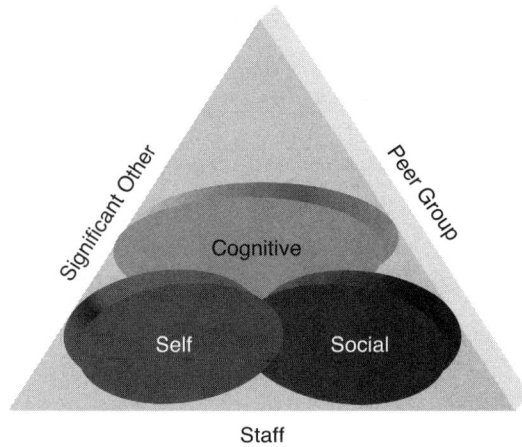

Figure 3.1.

Main elements of a treatment cycle

Members of the professional staff interchangeably perform all the program tasks: They evaluate, supervise, "coach" patients during remedial training "exercises," conduct groups or "community" activities, and provide personal counseling to the patients and their significant others. (Counseling assignments are also made by staff consensus.)

Experience, over many years, has shown that a patient-to-staff ratio of 2:1 is optimal in this setting. (Students who participate in internships or externships frequently make it possible to have a staff-to-patient ratio of nearly 1:1.)

Patients as a Peer Group. Within the treatment cycle, 13 to14 individuals who qualify for this type of program, form a peer group. Members of the peer group support, critique, inspire, and serve as role models for each other.

They range in age from 19 to 60 years; have varied educational backgrounds (ranging from high school graduates to people with college and postgraduate forms of education), have different life experiences (ranging from single young adults to married individuals with children), and have varied work and professional experiences (ranging from young people whose pursuit of their career goals was interrupted by the brain injury to people who had achieved successful professional or business careers before their brain injury).

Significant Others as Active Participants. On any given day, half of the patient peer group's significant others are present at the program. The significant others are active participants in all the program activities. Under the guidance of the professional staff, they provide feedback, assume role-playing assignments, and represent to the patient peer group excellent models of mature, well-behaved, and empathic individuals. By their deferential (i.e., respectful) and appreciative attitude toward the professional staff, the significant others inspire the patient peer group to adopt the same attitude.

Treatments Address Multiple Inadequacies Simultaneously. If at all possible, the treatments should address multiple inadequacies of the patients simultaneously in a coordinated and complementary fashion. As indicated in Figure 3.1, the program addresses in an integrated fashion interventions that are aimed at dealing with the personal disturbances (e.g., problems with the "injured sense of self"), the cognitive impairments, and the interpersonal (i.e., social) impairments of the patients.

Benefits of a Structured "Therapeutic Community"

The "therapeutic community" type of program is a powerful clinical "tool" for facilitating the processes that lead to compensation for deficits that have resulted from the brain injuries. Figure 3.2 indicates the main benefits of this therapeutically structured milieu.

The *structured nature* of the daily program schedule and the remedial interventions produce a sense of familiarity. In a matter of days, the familiarity breeds comfort by helping the patients to anticipate of "what is to come." (This, however, is more implicit in the case of patients with impaired memory.) Familiarity thus produces a feeling of "safety," because—under these conditions—the chances for the occurrence of a failure to cope are significantly diminished.

Through *awareness and understanding*, feeling "safe" makes it possible to motivate the patient to participate in the program and helps the patient

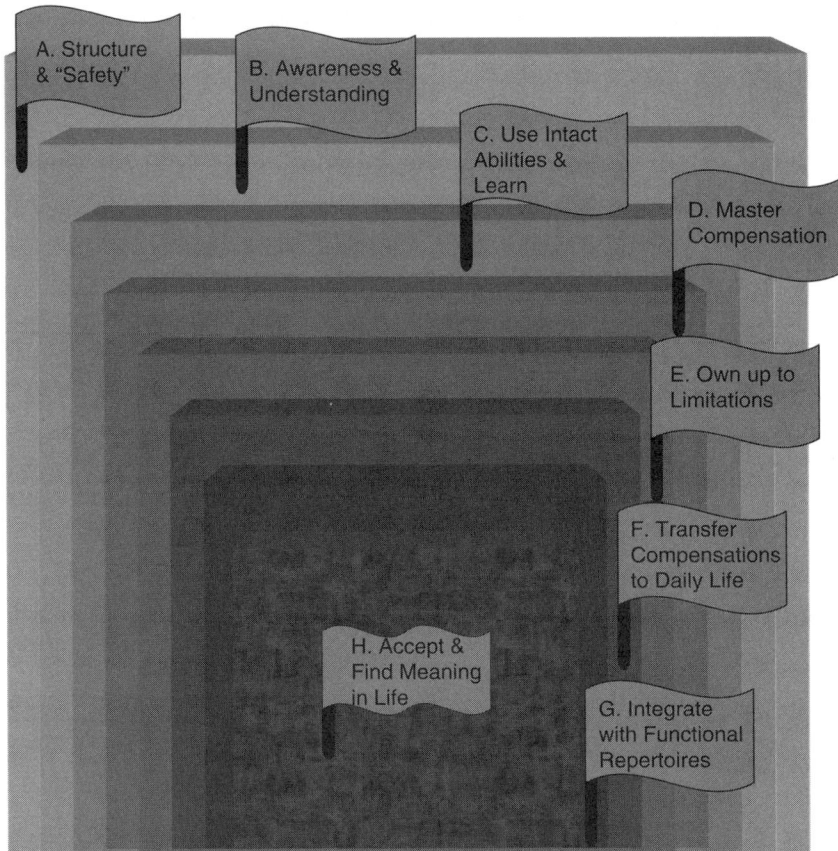

Figure 3.2.

The benefits of a therapeutic milieu program structure

to understand the need for systematic rehabilitative activities. What at first seems irrelevant and difficult becomes meaningful and doable.

Beginning to use still *intact abilities facilitates the learning process*. Since the "danger" of experiencing catastrophic response is significantly lessened, the "organismic defense" is no longer "needed." The person can, therefore, begin (once again) to learn and establish a knowledge base (i.e., to acquire compensatory skills). The learning of skills depends on the level or zone of potential development, which varies from individual to individual. This zone, therefore, defines the level of skill, or task complexity, that can be mastered by a given individual. Thus, with practice the person can move from his or her initial (baseline) ability to his or her potential level of attainment.

Mastery of compensatory skills helps to increase confidence. Confidence, slowly replaces defensiveness and permits the person (under guided conditions) to move forward to meet challenges that previously were easy to address, but now seem too difficult to face.

With the *improved ability to cope* (and the realization that he or she can still learn new things), the patient will gradually begin to exhibit the "moral courage" that is necessary for acknowledging (i.e., owning up to) limitations that the brain injury caused.

Learned compensatory skills and "strategies" can now begin to be applied by the patient in his or her daily life outside of the program, with the urging and with the needed assistance of the staff and the significant others.

With *sufficient practice of the compensatory skills (or strategies)*—learned in the program and applied away from the program—the chances are enhanced that both habituation the rendering of compensatory skills into semiautomatic behavioral routines) and integration (of the newly learned compensatory skills with the person's other, intact, functional repertoires) will occur.

Given these conditions, experience has shown that patients are ready to *accept their disability* and can go on finding *meaning in their life after rehabilitation.*

The Cumulative Effect of Multidimensional Interventions

In the "therapeutic community" structure of the holistic program—the cumulative effects of daily complementary and mutually reinforcing cognitive, therapeutic, clinical management, and "community" intervention—a gradual transformation is produced in the brain-injured individual over the duration of a treatment cycle. From an initial dysfunctional and despairing state of mind, the individual can slowly move toward becoming a compensated, functionally competent, interpersonally better adjusted, and self-accepting person. Changes occur within the limits of the current capacities and the individual's ultimate potential to readapt following the brain injury. Figure 3.3 depicts this process. In the following sections, each aspect is briefly described.

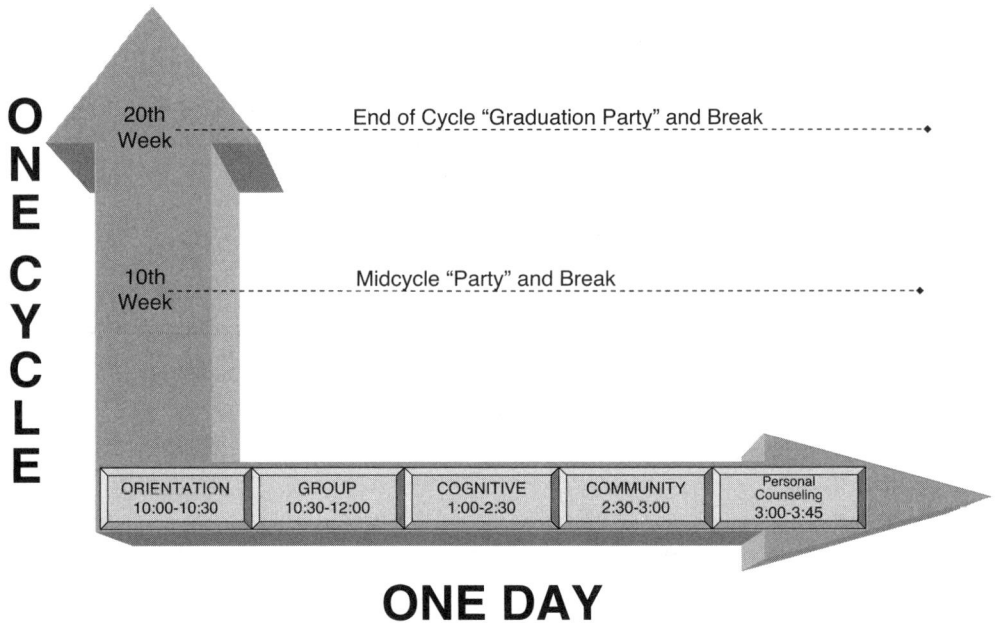

ONE DAY

| ORIENTATION 10:00-10:30 | GROUP 10:30-12:00 | COGNITIVE 1:00-2:30 | COMMUNITY 2:30-3:00 | Personal Counseling 3:00-3:45 |

20th Week — End of Cycle "Graduation Party" and Break

10th Week — Midcycle "Party" and Break

Figure 3.3.

Cumulative effects of complementary remedial, therapeutic, and "community" activities

Coordinated Treatments: One Day in the Program

In the following sections, each of the treatment components as they unfold in a typical program day and throughout the entire cycle are briefly described.

Orientation

Each program day begins with the assembly of the entire group of trainees, the significant others present during that given day, and the clinical staff who are assigned to lead the orientation session. This small-group procedure is designed to establish continuity; teach the trainees how to set realistic remedial goals (for a day, for a week, for a weekend, and for longer periods); promote the use of compensatory props and compensatory strategies; and foster willingness on the part of the trainees to assess their progress and difficulties in the presence of their peers, staff, and significant others. At the beginning of each cycle, based on the results of the initial assessment, the clinical team prepares a poster for each trainee. This poster identifies for the trainee the first core cognitive or neurobehavioral problem that, in the opinion of the staff, must be ameliorated by the trainee, so that meaningful progress will become possible in the remedial process. Outlined on this poster are the problem (e.g., "Dysinhibition, manifested as impulsivity"); the solution sought (e.g., "Become a deliberate preplanner and thoughtful responder"); and a four- to five-step operational action sequence or "strategy", describing how the trainee can ameliorate the problem.

These posters are presented to one trainee at a time, each morning, in the presence of the entire community. The presentation and the dialogue with the trainee receiving the poster are videotaped. Once the logic underlying the staff's selection of the particular problem and the method for ameliorating it are explained to the trainee, he or she is asked to restate the message on the poster in his or her own words. The trainee is then asked to endorse (or reject) the staff's recommendation. The trainee is also asked to assert his or her willingness to work toward ameliorating (i.e., improving) the deficient areas. The poster is then hung on the wall, in full view of the community, and remains there throughout the treatment cycle. This procedure is repeated until each trainee's personal poster is presented. Thus, all trainees and significant others can appreciate, at a glance, the particular problem that each trainee must learn to compensate for, as a first clinical priority.

Interpersonal Group Exercises

This individualized daily exercise is conducted in the presence of the therapeutic community. It is designed to improve interpersonal communication skills, malleability, and self-acceptance. The exercises consist of a series of rehabilitation-relevant themes that serve as the vehicles for the attainment of various clinical psychotherapeutic goals. Trainees—the patients—gradually learn how to acknowledge and speak about their losses in the cognitive, social, and vocational domains, while also regaining their sense of self-worth and dignity. The daily interpersonal group exercises are paradigmatic in nature. They are based on a set pattern of themes that differ from one another in the level of difficulty, from both the cognitive and emotional standpoints. Each of these themes lends itself to modifications as needed to suit particular clinical situations. Table 3.1 presents a list of these themes and provides a phenomenological analysis of the level of difficulty each poses to the trainee (i.e., the patient).

Each trainee on the "hot seat" is coached by a staff member. At the end of the exercise, the trainee receives organized feedback from the entire community about how effectively ideas were formulated and presented, the adequacy of the interpersonal communication style, and the manner in which guidance ("coaching") was accepted. The trainees who observe and give feedback to the person on the hot seat at the conclusion of the exercise are also coached on how to adequately analyze a peer's presentation and how to provide constructive criticism in an appropriate manner.

Once the program cycle is a few days "old," patients are persuaded not to decline participating in any of the group "exercises." The result is that when these "templates" become part of his or her behavioral repertoire, the trainee's mental outlook will have improved.

Trainees who are returning for an additional intensive remedial cycle undergo such "exercises" (training sessions in the therapeutic community program are called "exercises") that are specially modified to systematically address remaining problems in awareness, malleability, acceptance, or the style of the person's interpersonal communications. In the more advanced versions of these paradigmatic group exercises, typically two trainees are paired and helped by staff coaches to interview each other according to predetermined themes and procedures. Through such carefully orchestrated dialogues, calibrated according to the specific intellectual and emotional capabilities, trainees are guided by the staff to encourage, gently challenge, and support each other in the difficult process of coming to terms with their existential situation.

Peer Lunch

Trainees are encouraged to take their lunch hour with peers and those significant others who are present. This informal interpersonal hour

Table 3.1. A List of Themes for the Daily Interpersonal Group Exercises, in a Given Treatment Cycle

Description of assignment (i.e., of the theme)	Phenomenological analysis by level of cognitive-emotional difficulty of the assignment
1. Introduce yourself	(a) From among the many biographical facts, patient must select those facts with which he/she wishes to introduce himself/herself. (b) Plan how to present them to the audience.
2. Describe an accomplishment in your life, before the injury, that pleased you to have achieved. (Accomplishment could be objective and could have been achieved during one's early childhood, or during adulthood.)	(a) Think back about trainee's accomplishments. (b) Select the one that pleases him or her most to have achieved. (c) Plan how to present it to the audience.
3. Describe a personality quality of yours that you appreciate having.	(a) Introspect, focusing on personality qualities he or she possesses. (b) Select the one that pleases him or her to have. (c) Plan how to present it to the audience.
4. Tell a peer (of your choice) which of his or her personality qualities you came to appreciate or respect.	(a) Decide which of his or her peers to invite. (b) Reflect on that peer's personality qualities. (c) Select the one quality that the trainee respects most. (d) Plan how to present his or her impression to the person that he or she selected.
5. Describe a personality quality you possess that will prevent you from becoming a "bitter and defeated" person in the future.	(a) Introspect, focusing on his or her personality qualities that could help prevent "bitterness and a sense of defeat." (b) Select the one that he or she considers to be the most helpful. (c) Plan how to present it to the audience.
6. Make believe (imagine) that you are a junior member of this program's staff. With the help of a senior supervisor (who will be your coach) interview yourself—as role played by your personal counselor—about your progress so far, and what remains, still, for you to achieve so that your rehabilitation will be successful.	(a) Assume the mental attitude of a junior staff member (i.e., an "other"). (b) Adopt the mind-set of an objective, but empathic, professional. (c) Sustain over the duration of the exercise the role he or she has adopted. (d) Maintain, throughout, an "open," calm, receptive, and rational mode of thinking (instead of becoming overwhelmed by emotions upon hearing what his or her "ego other" has to say).

provides trainees with an opportunity to practice communication and socialization skills in a naturalistic setting. Trainees are encouraged to invite prospective candidates, who are undergoing assessment, to take lunch with them. Members of the staff are not, as a rule, included in these peer lunches.

Individualized Cognitive Remedial Training

Individualized cognitive-remedial training exercises are carried out in accordance with a preset curriculum and are tailored to each trainee's unique constellation of deficits. Thus, trainees are clinically matched, each day, with one or two of their peers to perform (according to their respective treatment plans and under the guidance of a staff coach) cognitive exercises designed to ameliorate difficulties in: initiating purposeful activities or ideas; controlling impulsive behaviors; focusing attention on a specific task by "screening out" internal or external distractions and sustaining their concentration for the required durations; effectively processing visual-perceptual and spatial-motor information; and using higher-level (convergent, divergent, and executive) reasoning.

The individualized cognitive-remedial training sessions are conducted in a manner that integrates three cardinal principles: (1) The cognitive training is executed hierarchically, focusing initially on the amelioration of basic attentional functions and ending with the remediation of higher-level logical reasoning deficits. (2) The training is conducted according to the principle of "saturation cuing," whereby the trainee is initially provided with maximum cues (or receives demonstrations of how to perform tasks in the most optimal fashion). Gradually the trainee receives fewer and fewer cues, until he or she achieves mastery of the training task. Successful mastery of a training procedure is demonstrated when the trainee can perform that procedure adequately, unaided by others, any time after mastery has taken place. Included in the principle of saturation cuing is the notion of "habituation" (i.e., a newly acquired compensatory skill must be practiced until it becomes a semiautomatic behavioral procedure). (3) The third principle is that a newly mastered compensatory skill must be applied in as many real-life situations as possible in order to become part of the trainee's functional repertoire.

It is important in this context to also point out that a distinction must be made between the meaning of the concepts of generalization and transfer of learning. In our experience, it is not realistic to expect true generalization of learned compensations. Rather, the practical goal should be to achieve a transfer of learning (from the compensatory training situation to real-life situations) that can be attained only through repeated applications, in a variety of functional contexts.

Community Hour

This daily group exercise is conducted with the participation of a full "community." It is designed to: (1) foster a sense of "citizenship" and group belonging; (2) improve social appropriateness of behavior; (3) enhance the trainee's willingness and ability to comply with socially acceptable rules of conduct; and (4) promote a sense of competence and a reconstituted sense of self. With the entire community seated in a large circle, each day, one of the trainees is selected to chair the session. Typically, one question, which has been prepared in advance of the daily community hour, is raised. The question is written down by the trainees who proceed to prepare, in writing, a concise and well-targeted response to that question. Then, each trainee in turn is called on by the chair to articulate, in front of the community, his or her response. Others (e.g., staff, significant others, and visitors) are then called on by the chair to comment. The sources of these questions vary. Often they are raised by one member of the staff, with the foreknowledge and agreement of the others. At other times, a particular trainee will ask a question that the trainee discussed and rehearsed with his or her personal counselor. Occasionally, a significant other, or a visitor, will pose a question.

While the questions vary, they are designed to provide the trainees with repeated experiences in articulating their ideas in front of their peers and hearing what others have to say on the same topic. The topics of the questions that are discussed during the "community" hour deal with issues such as the need to accept one's disability with "calm dignity," the rationale for rehabilitative training procedures, and the desirability of finding meaning in one's life following rehabilitation, despite the restrictions that have been imposed by the brain injury. The frequent presence of visiting professionals from different countries also provides excellent opportunities for trainees to "think on their feet" and to "teach" the visitors about particular facets of the program. Thus, the cumulative effects of chairing the sessions, responding effectively to challenging questions, and explaining program elements to visiting professionals bolsters (i.e., supports) the building-up of the trainee's self-esteem and confidence. An additional function of the "community" session is provided by the fact that as they advance in the treatment cycle, trainees are helped to formulate and pose challenging and controversial rehabilitation-relevant questions to their peers, thereby increasing their ability to deal with the "give and take" of real-life social situations. For example, a common question is: "Do you tell people about your brain injury?"

Personal Counseling

The trainee meets with his or her personal counselor at a minimum of twice a week. The counseling sessions are designed to help the trainee understand the overall program objectives, in terms that are relevant to his or her individual needs; develop the necessary rapport with the counselor, so that the counselor may serve as the trainee's "ombudsperson"; coach the trainee on how to optimally implement compensatory strategies and techniques; foster (in the more reticent or socially isolated trainee) a sufficient degree of confidence to bring relevant personal concerns to the therapeutic community; and help the trainee to transfer gains made in the program to the home environment. Personal counseling is viewed as an adjunct to the broader behavior-shaping activities and psychotherapeutic influences engendered by other program activities.

Trainees (and their significant others) often hear the staff telling them that the process of compensation and the transformation of an individual from a dysfunctional and despairing state of mind to the level of maximum functional competence possible and self-acceptance, is a slow, laborious, and often painful process. Figure 3.4 illustrates this "spiral-like" process.

Accordingly, when the individual is initially in a despairing (often also agitated) state of mind, he or she must first be helped to become willing and able to engage in the process of rehabilitation. If the brain injury is also characterized by restlessness, and impulsivity, or it's opposite, the

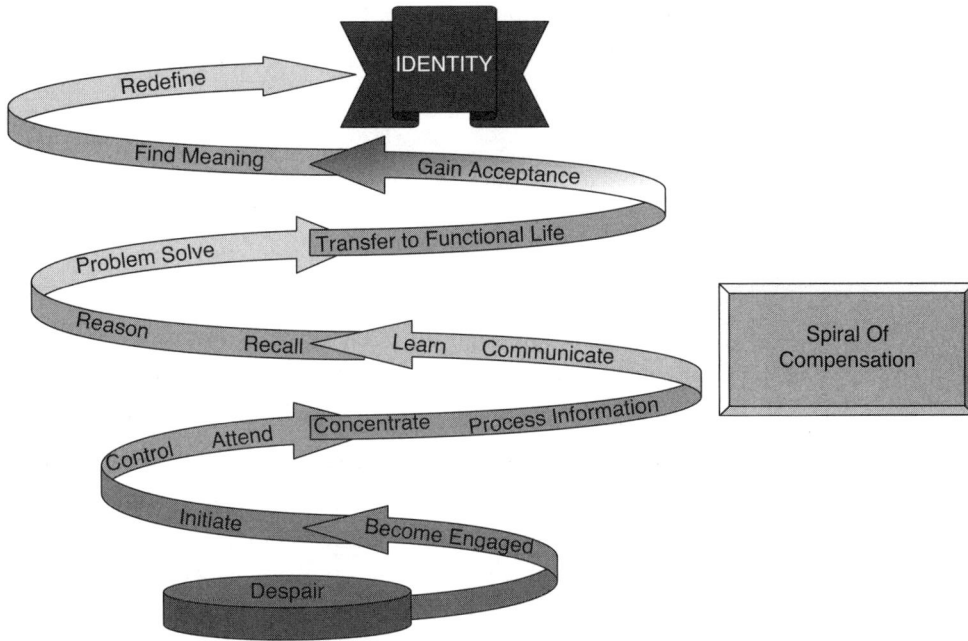

Figure 3.4.

The unfolding of the compensatory process

inability to initiate and persist at purposeful behaviors, these must be handled effectively, before it becomes possible to improve the person's attention and concentration. In other words, the brain-injured individual must achieve first the qualities of a "student", before he or she can be expected to engage in effective learning processes. Once the person is ready to engage in learning activities, the remedial training can focus on helping the individual to compensate for deficits in the area of (verbal and visual) information processing, in the area of interpersonal communications, in the area of learning and recalling new information, and in the area of higher level reasoning. Once the person has mastered (i.e., learned) how to implement compensatory skills, it is necessary to habituate (i.e., make them semiautomatic parts of one's behavior) so that they would become integrated with the person's other functional repertoires.

Experience has shown that only after brain-injured people achieve success in compensating for deficits do their morale improve and self-acceptance follow. But, we have also learned that to attain such transformation the individuals must possess certain personality characteristics (the study of which is presently the focus of intensive clinical research).

Counseling for the Family Significant Others

The personal counselor who is assigned to each trainee meets 1 to 2 hours per week with the trainee's family, or the significant others, either individually or jointly, as clinically indicated. The therapeutic approach with family or significant others is principally psychoeducational in nature. It is designed to provide the significant others with the necessary education concerning the nature and functional consequences of the brain injury of their loved one, and the understanding of the purposes and possibilities of rehabilitation; as well as the skills and emotional supports they will require to be able to cope effectively with their respective trainees and the changed family and social roles that will result from the injury of their loved one. The process often involves the need for making painful decisions.

Weekly and Multiple-Family Group Sessions for Significant Others

The significant others and family members of all the trainees meet once each week for a 1½ hour multiple-family group session. These sessions are not attended by the trainees. The meetings (a combination of lectures, presentations, and group discussions) are focused around a core curriculum that parallels the educational process of the trainees. These include topics concerning awareness and understanding of the nature of the brain injury; issues relating to malleability and coaching; questions about how best to help their loved one implement compensations they are being taught in the program (i.e., how to facilitate their transfer to the home environment); and, finally, questions concerning acceptance of the permanence of the brain injury and its future personal, social, and vocational implications. Significant others are also provided with guidelines for managing (in the parlance of the program, "coaching") the trainee at home. They are also helped to develop an in-depth understanding of the purpose, techniques, and outcomes that each can realistically expect from their loved one.

Ad Hoc Crisis Interventions and Clinical Management Sessions

During any treatment cycle, a trainee and his or her significant others may meet with the clinical team for special "poster" sessions. These poster sessions are designed to provide optimal clinical "leverage", to make possible the desired modification in the trainee's attitude and behavior, and to form a therapeutic alliance between the trainee's significant others and the staff. These sessions are called "poster" sessions because the staff employs large colorful posters on which the problem and suggested solutions are outlined. Each poster session is videotaped to provide an audiovisual record for the trainee and significant others to review at home.

Coordinated Clinical Interventions at Mid-cycle and End of Treatment Cycle

Midcycle "Party"

By week 10 in the cycle, the trainees prepare (with the help of their personal coach) a carefully written and well-rehearsed formal presentation to an audience consisting of families, friends, and invited others (including former trainees and their families). Although the audience is "friendly" and a number of its constituent members are often familiar to the trainees, it nevertheless represents the "outside world" to them. The presentations are videotaped and subsequently are used in individual counseling or small-group sessions to enhance the trainee's awareness and acceptance. Participation in the preparation and delivery of the presentations is compulsory, as is the need for each trainee to accept the clinical inputs and editorial suggestions provided by the staff during the preparation of the speeches.

During the midcycle presentation, each trainee is required to deliver a brief and carefully edited didactic speech describing a particular facet of the program, such as its philosophy, the purpose of the interpersonal group exercises, the role of cognitive remediation, and the benefits of significant others in program participation. Following the didactic presentations, trainees deliver a personal statement as well. These statements describe their deficits, as they have come to understand them, as well as the progress they have been making in rehabilitation. For many, the midcycle party is the first public admission that they have sustained a brain injury, which has produced intellectual or behavioral limitations, and that these problems necessitate intensive remedial training, as well as the need to "gracefully" accept assistance from others. This public "owning" or admitting prepares the way for further progress in awareness and malleability. The fact that the personal speeches are well-rehearsed presentations that are much appreciated by the audience, ensures that the trainees experience their public disclosures as ego enhancing. The applause and the respect paid by the audience also enhance the trainees' self-confidence and self-acceptance.

The purpose of the midcycle "party" is to test how well the individual trainee has assimilated the various (personalized) rehabilitative interventions during his or her first 10 weeks in the program.

Although the midcycle party is the most prominent, even dramatic, event in the program (by virtue of the fact that the trainees, as a group, acting under the leadership of a master of ceremonies, one of their own, deliver a series of well-rehearsed speeches in front of an audience), it is an integral part of the treatments. It is the culmination of a process that has several preparatory aspects and several follow-up aspects, all of which are aimed at enhancing the individual trainee's self-confidence and self-esteem. The following clinical "landmarks" can be identified in this process:

1. The staff—acting as a "clinical council"—decides on which specific tasks should be assigned to each individual trainee. This also includes the decision of what should be the "talking points" the trainee should include in his or her speech.

2. The personal counselor will have to persuade the trainee to endorse the staff's suggested "talking points" and "work through" with the trainee how to put in the trainee's own written words the suggested talking points.

3. Once a speech is written, it then must be edited down to a 300-word coherent "speech."

4. The trainee group, then, rehearses together the delivery of the speeches. During these rehearsals, trainees receive concrete

suggestions as to how to deliver their speeches (e.g., what body language or tone of voice to use) to render them most effective and engaging.

5. Prior to the party itself, each trainee, states—in the presence of the peers—how he or she wishes to be perceived by the audience. (These wished-for impressions are written down on colorful posters and serve as part of the postparty self-critiques and feedback sessions.)

6. The actual presentations at the "party" are videotaped.

7. Following the "party," the personal statement of each trainee is viewed again and critiqued by all members of the "therapeutic community" (including visiting professionals or prospective program candidates who are present).

8. Lessons learned from these postparty critiques are "worked through" during the ensuing personal counseling sessions.

Although the audience, in front of which the presentations are made, is known to be "friendly," it nevertheless represents the "outside world." For most trainees, the personal speech (which includes explicit descriptions of the cognitive and behavioral deficits that have resulted from their brain injuries) is the first "public" admission that they sustained a brain injury that necessitates intensive rehabilitation and the "graceful" acceptance of help. This public "owning" (delivered in a calm and dignified manner) is much appreciated by the audience. This positive response enhances the trainee's ego and self-esteem, helping to motivate the individual to accept further rehabilitative interventions.

While the trainee's participation in the preparations and the delivery of the assigned speeches is expected, based on the "contractual" understanding between the trainee and the program staff, if a trainee is unhappy with, or refuses to accept, the suggested "talking points," he or she is allowed not to join the peers in their presentations. The trainee, in that case, will have to sit as part of audience and observe his or her peers "perform" on the stage. But not before the meaning of this "exemption" and its implication is discussed, privately, with the counselor or the program director. The following case illustrates such an intervention. ("Natasha")

Natasha was a 26-year-old young woman who, at age 6, came to the United States from Russia with her parents. She was a problem child since her early childhood: She was socially isolated because of constant fights with her peers and made a poor adjustment as a student throughout the primary and high school years. Natasha's problematic adjustment, however, was not due to a lack of intelligence but, primarily, because of her constant conflicts with her teachers and other authority figures. Her rebellious behavior at school was merely an extension of her problems with her parents at home. Natasha constantly defied her parents, ran away from home often, and "could not be reasoned with," according to her parents. She nevertheless graduated from high school and enrolled at a small college in another state. After a similarly eventful 4 years, Natasha graduated from college with a B.A. degree in communications. But she was unable to hold down, for any length of time, any of a number of jobs, had several "run-ins" with the law, and lost her only male friend. All of Natasha's difficulties could be attributed to her aggressive, authority-defying style of communication, her "thin skin" (she was ever-ready to become "insulted" by even mildly critical comments), and her extreme self-righteousness.

At the age of 23, Natasha became suddenly ill. She was flown home by her parents (both of whom are research scientists employed by a drug company). In New York, Natasha underwent an emergency neurosurgical procedure. A large brain tumor was removed from the frontotemporal region of her brain. Following the neurosurgical intervention, Natasha exhibited many cognitive deficits and her already problematic behaviors became exacerbated. She clearly presented a major challenge to the doctors and therapists who tried to manage her.

In February of 2008, Natasha was evaluated by our program. She was accepted for a 6-week probationary period. Our understanding with Natasha and her parents was that she would have to comply with all of our staff's requests, abide by the "rules of the house," and show tangible evidence that the treatments she received in our program would gradually improve both her cognitive functions as well as her interpersonal behaviors (including her relationships with her parents).

Although, Natasha was a difficult trainee, she worked hard and enjoyed her membership in our "therapeutic community." She responded acceptably to the firm, but respectful, approach by the staff, quickly realizing that compliance with the rules and appropriate behavior on her part resulted in social acceptance, respect, and empathic responses by her peers and the staff alike. (Natasha craved the respect of others and proved willing to work toward earning it.)

In the eighth week of the program, Natasha, like her peers, received her two assigned speeches, which were to be delivered during the midcycle party. Her first assignment was to speak about "the philosophy of the program," and the second assignment was to deliver a personal statement. Natasha felt "honored" by the philosophy assignment and cooperated eagerly with her counselor in crafting her speech (according to the "talking points" that were given to her for this speech). However, she was very unhappy and actively expressed her resentment for "not being allowed" to say what she was "prepared to say" in front of the audience about her personal progress in the program. This prompted a private conversation between Natasha and the program director. (Her personal counselor was also present during this discussion.) The following points summarize what transpired during this session (D. is shorthand for director; N. for Natasha):

a. D. told N. that the staff was concerned about the fact that "you are unhappy about having to prepare your personal speech following our suggested talking points."

b. N. responded in an irritable tone: "You promised to respect us and not to boss us." She then demanded to know: "Why can't I say things my own way?"

c. D. told N. that he felt sad that "you interpret the talking points as a form of bossing." But, D. added, "This is not the way we, the staff, see things. We promised to treat you with respect and we have kept our promise. Treating someone with respect also means telling the person the truth, with compassion. And the truth is that when you entered our program you also promised to trust us to guide you and help you become the competent and respected person you always wished to be. That promise included following our advice, even if initially it did not make sense to you."

d.   But N. was in no mood to listen. In an agitated state, she jumped up from her chair and shouted: "You guys are trying to shove down my throat *your* words!" (referring to the talking points).

e.   Realizing N.'s agitation, D., in a calm and measured tone, said to N.: "Let me suggest that you think things over. If by tomorrow you will still feel uncomfortable working with G. (her counselor) on your personal speech, along the lines that we suggested, feel free to sit this one out. You will not deliver any speeches. You will sit in the audience and watch your peers perform on the stage. Let us know what you have decided to do by tomorrow." One hour later, Natasha returned and apologized for her outburst. She told the director that she decided to work on her speech with her counselor.

Midcycle Break

Following the review and critique of their midcycle presentations, the trainees and their significant others undergo (individualized) preparations for the 10-day midcycle break from the program. The purposes of the midcycle break are to test the ability of trainees:

a.   To function without the structure of the daily program in their naturalistic setting;

b.   To reintegrate them within their respective family structures;

c.   To test their willingness and ability to accept coaching, or assistance, from their significant others.

End-of-Cycle "Party"

At the end of the 20-week treatment cycle, each trainee receives an oral report card from the staff in the presence of the entire "community." Following the oral "report card," preparations for writing the end-of-cycle party speech begin. The process is quite similar to the one involving the midcycle party presentations. Once again, the staff prepares the "talking points" for each trainee.

Volume 3 of Chapter 3 DVD, Disc B presents two end-of-cycle speeches. (See "Ruth" further below and "Laura" in Chapter 5).

Case Study: "Ruth"

Ruth was a 53-year-old French teacher at a well-known high school. She had the reputation of being a dedicated, creative, hardworking, and tireless teacher. She spent long hours on planning—in great detail—every "encounter" she had with her students. Nothing was left to chance or to spontaneous improvisation. Although in her manner and tone she was always the "teacher," Ruth was also known to be a caring person. She was described by an astute (and admiring) colleague as being "a very attractive, obsessive-compulsive type of person, whose personality combined with her erudition and intellectual brilliance to make her the master teacher" she was.

Ruth's "minor" head injury was the result of horseplay between two of her students. She was hit on her head by a schoolbag full of books, which one student flung at the other. Although she never lost consciousness, this incident had resulted in diffuse brain impairments. Our comprehensive neuropsychological evaluation revealed that Ruth had sustained diffuse axonal injury (DAI) with a number of cognitive and neurobehavioral sequelae (attentional deficits; emotional lability; difficulty to modulate the expression of her feelings with a tendency to "catastrophize"; some problems with memory; and circumscribed problems in the domain of her higher level reasoning, particularly her executive functions). Our evaluation also suggested that Ruth's organically based problems were exacerbated by psychologically based symptoms of decompensation (in this previously well-adjusted individual with obsessive-compulsive personality features).

Ruth was examined by the neurologist who was employed by her school system and was declared "fit," to return immediately to her teaching duties. This neurologist rejected our well-documented neuropsychological findings as well as the recommendation that she enroll into our intensive day program. For, in his opinion, she was an "agitated," "suspicious," "dramatizer," and "manipulator" who (he clearly insinuated) was motivated by a desire to obtain financial gains from her injury. This neurologist did not know that several weeks later a PET scan, ordered by another neurologist, would corroborate our neurodiagnostic impressions. PET, (Position Emission Tomography) is a neuro-radiologic procedure which details abnormalities in cellular activity).

Thus, despite the demand by Ruth's school superintendent that she return to her teaching job, she enrolled in our program, at her own expense, leaving the task of a legal battle with her school system to her attorney.

Ruth's two treatment cycles at our facility, which spanned one full year, were very eventful. From the very start, she had a great deal of difficulty becoming a "student." Her tendency to frequently experience mentally "paralyzing" neurofatigue, to react in an irritable and poorly modulated manner (she became "insulted" and irritated by even "routine," or casual, corrective comments by our staff members and did not hesitate to express her displeasure) by voicing her negative thoughts (of the "what if" variety), to experience memory lapses and interferences with reasoning functions, to display poor morale and a pessimistic outlook on the future all rendered her a very challenging program trainee.

Gradually, however, Ruth came around. Aided by some of her positive personality characteristics and her intelligence, she:

- *Acquired an intellectual understanding of the true nature of her deficits and their functional implications;*

- *Showed that she had the potential to, ultimately, "make peace" with her predicament and her life after rehabilitation, even though, as she gradually came to understand, that life after rehabilitation would, in all probability, be different from her preinjury life.*

After a year of "negotiations" with her school district (which, in the meantime, became aware that, in case of a trial, Ruth would be represented by an array of renowned medical and neuropsychological experts), Ruth was offered an attractive proposal for an out-of-court settlement. The settlement was conditioned on her returning to her school for about 1 year. Then, Ruth would be able to retire from teaching with a generous lifetime pension. During her last year at her school, Ruth would be performing "light duties" (which she was perfectly able to perform in our program). Fortunately, by this time, Ruth already achieved the psychological transformation that was necessary to ensure that her postrehabilitation adjustment could be optimal.

After a year's work, final preparations for Ruth's graduation speech were under way. With several personal counseling sessions under her belt, Ruth was asked to put down in writing her personal assessment of how close she was to accepting and facing the future with the equanimity that would be necessary to find meaning in her life "after rehabilitation and retirement." As usual, her counselor gave her many specific questions to contemplate as she wrote down her thoughts and feelings. She was told by her counselor not to worry about the number of words, and that the "editing job, to a 300-word speech, will be done by you later, as an exercise in applying cognitive strategies that you have learned to improve your convergent *and* divergent *reasoning abilities as well as your* executive *functions."*

Ruth produced a four-page written document (about 1850 words), which is presented below in its entirety. (Bracketed comments are ours.)

> *At this point in my rehabilitation, I have become aware of my deficits and how they interact with each other. What I find myself thinking is that I need to have a continuous awareness, as I am still vulnerable to thinking, "why have I had to alter my life so radically, when I am feeling well and capable right now?" I am starting to make progress in that when I have these ideas, I remember, "yes, I have felt this way before," only to be suddenly reminded of my neurofatigue, how quickly it can surface and how debilitating it can be. I also keep in mind the feelings [that] I had while [I engaged in exercises of] "teaching" in the program. It was difficult [for me] to concentrate on the "the student" meaning [i.e., how they understood what I meant to say] if I was fatigued or if the student was unclear, or both. These thoughts are helping me to reach a more continuous awareness so that I can guard against embarking [in the future] on pursuits which could lead to failure and frustration.*
>
> *I am aware [of] and understand my deficits fairly well, although there are times when I need reminders as I don't always see [things clearly] "in the moment." I now know that I am particularly subject to neurofatigue, which stops me in my tracks, and makes me incapable of performing mental or physical activities. At such times, I am not able to effectively interact with others, even if I'm keeping [my tendency to become irritable] at bay. My information processing which now is slowed and still, at times, inaccurate, my memory, and higher level*

reasoning, including executive functions, can all be affected by my neurofatigue. In addition, I can still show symptoms of disinhibition, as well as problems with attention and concentration. In order to avoid this pitfall, I'll need to build in breaks, or at the very least, allow myself to get the needed rest, in order to prevent these deficits from surfacing.

I now understand fully that my brain injury is permanent. There is no repair for damaged or non-functioning neurons. This is why it is paramount that I master and habituate my strategies, so that I can achieve as functional a level as possible for the rest of my life. By being attentive to my "strategies," I'll function optimally. This is essential to having a productive life.

When I started the program, I was not malleable. In fact, I was fairly proud of the fact [that I was perceived as not being malleable] because I didn't want anyone to alter me. I had always been extremely capable at managing my life and saw no reason why I would need to change. Numerous factors and encounters contributed to this lack of trust. These included my own assumptions, observations, and certain messages that I heard from staff members [which irritated me]. Although I had been an empathic person before my injury, I became totally self-absorbed afterwards. Ellen [her counselor] has explained that this is a common, typical occurrence after a brain injury. It took until roughly [the] mid-cycle of my first cycle, to become aware [that my thinking began to] shift and to see that I was gradually regaining the ability to look outward, due to the inspirational aspects of the program. Connecting with my peers and the significant others [also] made [easier] my existence in the program. As I saw their growth and hope and heard encouraging messages [from the staff] and concerns for my [own] progress, I realized I needed to change my approach. This factor, more than any other, kept me going, so that when I was ready, I was able to integrate staff messages and move forward in my rehabilitation. At this point, I deeply wanted to make the changes, so that I could make progress, but I felt as if I was fighting against some of my basic tendencies [that prevented me from following] the staff's suggestions. Ultimately, as I gained more equanimity, I was able to process [information] more ably, and could then institute some of the staff recommendations. This change became evident for the first time in the interpersonal exercise [in which I role-played being a member of the staff whose job was to interview me, as role-played by my counselor].

In the future, I will not be in the program; therefore, [I] will not have staff coaches, or the structure of the program, as built-in reminders. I'll need to remain open to Steve's [her husband] suggestions, and at times my sons', when they see an issue, differently than me when I am still not always able to because neurofatigue is overtaking me. When it comes to reasoning, I will need to remain open to consulting with Steve before sending out e-mails. Having a "trusted other's" opinion, makes me feel more certain that I'm putting "my best foot forward" and that I'm "coming across" the way I want to. By understanding that my deficits can appear precipitously, I must continue to seek the assistance which I know can benefit me. I recall during the first cycle when I voiced my concern that coaching would make me dependent, I [now know] that it would actually make me more independent or capable. With the various aspects of the program having its effects on me [or perhaps my becoming more able to implement the staff recommendations], I have seen how much more capable I have become in modulating my emotions, improving my interpersonal relationships, [as well as improving] information processing, and reasoning. I am sure there are more improvements that have taken place.

I am not yet certain whether or not I have mastered and habituated the necessary strategies in order to function optimally. There are times that I believe I must have habituated some of my strategies due to the fact that I am not aware that I am using them. Part of the definition of habituation [is] that one uses [compensatory] strategies so seamlessly that one is not aware of using them. They become semi-automatic. Perhaps this is why I have not been aware of precisely [which] strategies I'm using, and when.

Specifically speaking, I have become effective at delaying and considering what I will and won't say in most situations. Previous to regaining this ability, I had, at best little, and frequently, no control over what came out of my mouth. I feel as if I have become reliable at pre-empting this problem. (I have learned some important "lessons.")

Delaying [my response] can induce self-monitoring. But, there are numerous other situations in which I need to remind myself to self-monitor. If I'm feeling emotional, I need to step back and be objective in order to be sure I'm interpreting information accurately; so that, my decisions can be well reasoned. This could also be a good time to consult a trusted other, so that I'm getting another perspective, one that is truly objective.

I am aware that [at present] I verify more regularly, but am uncertain whether or not I have mastered this strategy. There are times when I notice that I have verified and other times when I realize I need to verify and then do so.

By remaining aware and frequently asking myself how I'm doing, I will be more vigilant and be able to prevent problems from occurring. I hope that by returning as a visitor to this program, I'll not only be able to help others, but also keep these strategies at the forefront of my mind.

When I first began in this program, I was fraught with worries. I almost said "full of fright". [I was] preoccupied [with thoughts of] getting back to my old life. I realize now that wanting to get back to the "old me" is very common for people with brain injuries. Witnessing dramatic changes, without understanding them or knowing how to improve one's functioning, can cause an individual to become obsessive, self-absorbed, and anxious. These emotional difficulties can have a bearing on behavior, and consequently (on) interpersonal relationships.

At this point in my rehabilitation, I have reached a point where I'm feeling calm and significantly more in control of my deficits. This makes it possible to accept the idea that I have "restrictions"—as Goldstein said—or limitations that I must willingly accept in order to function [at my best]. By accepting [the reality of] these limitations and viewing them as [the results of my injury] I will be able to be productive in life. This in turn will help me find meaning in my life.

Rehabilitation from brain injury is a life-long process, necessary because brain injury is permanent. By keeping my progress, compensatory strategies, and caveats in mind, I'll be able to achieve more successes in my pursuits. The satisfaction that I [will] derive [from such pursuits] will lead towards true self-acceptance.

Although I will not be able to continue formal rehabilitation within this program, I believe that the staff's recommendation will be for me to remain aware of the successes I've made and to keep in mind, or be vigilant of, the possible stumbling blocks [that] I can encounter. I am already aware that I will be welcome as a visitor, but perhaps, given some time and moving closer towards [my own] self-acceptance, I'll be encouraged to be a peer counselor [in this program] so that I can give back to others. Having reached a point where I can look backward and see how far I have come, can help me to encourage others in their own rehabilitation.

End-of-Cycle "Party"

At the end of the 20-week treatment cycle, each trainee receives an "oral report card" from the staff in the presence of the entire "community." These oral report cards are videotaped. The trainee receives an objective evaluation by the staff of his or her success, or failure, to achieve the clinical objectives that were formulated for him or her by the staff at the beginning of the treatment cycle. The trainee is then asked to explicitly express (1) his or her acceptance of the present existential situation, (2) the commitment to pursue the staff's recommendations, and (3) whether or not he or she has an optimistic outlook on the future.

Following the "oral report card," each trainee is asked to write a final 300 words "graduation" speech. (The clinical procedures for the preparation, rehearsal, and delivery of the end-of-cycle "graduation" speech, are similar to the preparation of the mid-cycle speeches).

End-of-Cycle Break

At the end-of-cycle party, all trainees—those who are finally discharged from the program as well as those who are expected to return for an

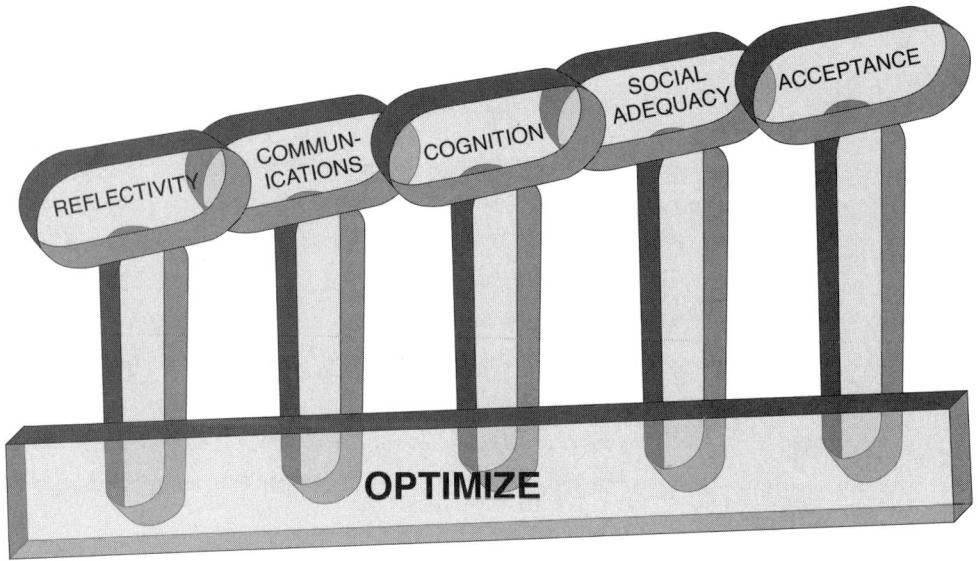

Figure 3.5.

The functional (outcome) objectives of neuropsychological rehabilitation

additional cycle—are prepared for the postparty break, which ranges from 3 to 6 weeks.

At home, each is carefully observed by the significant others to determine the degree to which each is able to adjust without the program structure and the peer group.

Figure 3.5 is a summary of the functional outcomes that are expected to result from the intensive remedial interventions.

The goals of the functional outcomes that result from a trainee's participation in the program are to regain the ability to reflect and deliberate; to become an effective communicator of his or her thoughts (and feelings); to optimize the ability to compensate for deficits in the cognitive area; to become, once again, socially adjusted; and to accept with equanimity and calmness one's existential situation (which includes an improved ego identity).

DVD Illustrations

Chapter 3 DVD, Volume 1

Sample 1: Orientation Session

Sample 2: Interpersonal Group Exercises

Sample 3: Cognitive Remedial Exercises

Sample 4: Community Session

Sample 5: Personal Counseling'

Chapter 3 DVD, Volume 2

Sample 1: Mid-cycle speech and post party critique

Sample 2: Speech editing

Sample 3: End-of-cycle speech

Suggested Readings

Ben-Yishay, Y. (1983). Cognitive remediation viewed from the perspective of a systematic clinical research program in rehabilitation. *Cognitive Rehabilitation*, *1*(5), 4–6.

Ben-Yishay, Y. (2000). Post acute neuropsychological rehabilitation. In A. L. Christensen & B. Uzzel (Eds.), *International handbook of neuropsychological rehabilitation* (pp. 127–135). New York: Kluwer.

Ben-Yishay, Y., & Diller, L. (1993). Cognitive remediation in traumatic brain injury: Update and issues. *Archives of Physical Medicine Rehabilitation 74*, 204–213.

Ben-Yishay, Y., Diller, L., Gerstman, L., & Gordon, W. (1970). Relationship between initial competence and ability to profit from cues in brain damaged individuals. *Journal of Abnormal Psychology*, *75*, 248–259.

Ben-Yishay, Y., Diller, L., & Mandleberg, I. (1970). Ability to profit from cues as a function of initial competence in normal and brain-injured adults: A replication of previous findings. *Journal of Abnormal Psychology, 76,* 378–379.

Ben-Yishay, Y., & Gold, J. (1990). Therapeutic milieu approach to neuropsychological rehabilitation. In R. L. Wood (Ed.) *Neurobehavioral sequelae of traumatic brain injury* (pp. 194–215). London: Taylor and Francis.

Ben-Yishay, Y., & Lakin, P. (1989). Structured group treatment for brain injury survivors. In D. W. Ellis & A. L. Christensen (Eds.), *Neuropsychological treatment after brain injury* (pp. 271–295). Boston: Kluwer.

Ben-Yishay, Y., Lakin, P., Ross, B., Rattok, J., Piasetsky, E. B., & Diller, L. (1983). Psychotherapy following severe brain injury: Issues and answers. *N.Y.U. Rehabilitation Monograph 66,* 128–148.

Ben-Yishay, Y., Rattok, J., Ross, B., Schaier, A. H., Scherzer, P., & Diller, L. (1979). Structured group techniques for heterogeneous groups of head trauma patients. *N.Y.U. Rehabilitation Monograph, 60,* 38–88.

Prigatano, G., & Ben-Yishay, Y. (1999). Psychotherapy and psychotherapeutic intervention. In M. Rosenthal (Ed.), *Rehabilitation of the adult and child with traumatic brain injury* (3rd ed., pp. 271–283). Philadelphia: F.A. Davis.

Ross, B., Ben-Yishay, Y., Lakin, P., Piasetsky, E. B., Rattok, J., & Diller, L. (1983). The role of family therapy in the treatment of the severely brain injured. *N.Y.U. Rehabilitation Monograph, 66,* 113–127.

Ross, B., Ben-Yishay, Y., Lakin, P., Rattok, J., Thomas, J. L., & Diller, L. (1982). Using a "therapeutic community" to modify the behavior of head trauma patients in rehabilitation. *N.Y.U. Rehabilitation Monograph, 66,* 84–112.

Chapter 4   *Assembling and Training the Professional Staff*

This chapter: (1) outlines the typical ways in which the professional staff functions in our "therapeutic community" setting; (2) identifies the temperamental and personality characteristics, as well as the clinical skills, that make a person best suited for team membership in this type of program; (3) illustrates—with DVD excerpts—how the staff deliberates while functioning as a "clinical council"; and (4) illustrates—with DVD excerpts—how a new candidate for staff membership is interviewed.

Typical Roles Played by the Staff

As is the case with the trainees and their significant others, the staff members in a "therapeutic community" function—and are perceived to function—as a united "coaching team." The term "coach" is borrowed from sports and complements the term "trainee." Both appellations are meant to suggest that the program is aimed at training individuals so they can gain optimal functioning, rather than be in a program designed to treat "patients."

In this setting, staff members do not work as "specialists." They are not involved, exclusively, as test administrators and interpreters, or as cognitive trainers, or as personal counselors. Instead, each member of the staff is trained and expected to perform all of these tasks, in addition to also serving as members of the "clinical council" (or the "coaching team"). Upon entering the program, trainees and their significant others (SOs) are told that (1) the program policies are the products of joint deliberations by the entire team; (2) training and counseling assignments are made on the basis of team consensus; (3) all remedial and therapeutic activities will be conducted according to an overall treatment plan that will be formulated by the program staff; and (4) acceptance of these terms are, in effect, part of the trainee's and SO's "contract" with the program.

In addition to these guidelines, the "contractual" agreement conveys: (1) that it will be the task of the program staff to define and clarify the boundaries between the topics that will be exclusively dealt with as private matters and topics that will be open for joint discussion during "community" or group procedures; (2) that each individual's personal dignity (including the freedom from being embarrassed) will be safeguarded; (3) that all the "community" members—including the trainees, their significant others, members of the staff (and even visitors to the program)—are expected to refrain from disclosing to "outsiders" any information concerning their peers or any deliberations that take place within the "community." For only in this way can the program participants feel "safe" and develop the required trust for wholehearted participation in the program.

Desirable Temperamental, Personality, and Clinical Skills of the Staff Members

Experience has shown that professionals who proved to be best suited for membership in a "therapeutic community" possess the following characteristics:

1. Temperamentally, they are energetic, even-tempered people, who can tolerate working effectively for many hours a day.

2. In terms of personality, they are able to project (i.e., to make others see them as having) personal warmth (without being "mushy" and overly emotional or sentimental) and are empathetic (i.e., are able to put themselves in the other person's "shoes").

3. In terms of the style of their communication, they should be plain speakers, refraining whenever possible from using technical jargon; be able to "project" sincerity; and be perceived as persons who enjoy helping others in need—but who also expect people to "stand on their own two feet" and help themselves, by finding

within themselves, the determination to do what they can to better their life.

4. As human beings, these staff members should have personal interests and hobbies that are not exclusively focused on their profession.

5. As members of the team, they should be seen as "natural" team players, who respect their colleagues; are willing and able to accept constructive criticisms; but who can also think independently. Persons who are best suited to be members of the team should also be known to reliably keep their promises and to adhere to the program policies.

6. In terms of their specific clinical skills and talents, members of the staff should be equally comfortable performing one-on-one types of remedial and therapeutic interventions as well as group or "community" types of interventions.

7. Finally, as members of the "clinical council," staff members should possess good analytic abilities—in other words, a capacity to see the underlying common causes of specific behaviors that are exhibited by a given trainee—and should be able to formulate specific, concrete, and operationalized approaches to implementing staff decisions. Likewise, they should possess the ability to express their opinion (during team deliberations) in a persuasive manner.

Selected Illustrations of How the Team Functions

Chairing Team Meetings. To ensure that all team members will be heard, on an equal footing with the senior staff, the following procedures have been adopted: (1) All members of the staff who wish to speak, including the senior staff, must be recognized by the designated team leader who chairs meetings. (The program director, or the senior staff, rarely, if ever, chairs the meetings.) (2) Once a person has the floor, no one is allowed to interrupt him or her without the chair's permission. (3) A speaker is expected to be as concise as possible; to stick to the issues under discussion; and to speak in plain, jargon-free English.

To train themselves to become effective team deliberators, members of the staff are encouraged to prepare in advance some written "talking points." Then, once they have the floor, they are encouraged to stick to these talking points (without digressions or improvisations). Members of the staff are also provided with written suggestions about how to behave during staff deliberations. The following examples are illustrative:

- When you wish to propose something, say: "I propose (such and such)"; then, say: "and here are my reasons why."

- Always *be explicit* when you wish to verify your understanding of what another team member has said. Also, be explicit when you wish to *agree* or *disagree* with part of, or the entire, statement of a colleague.

- Clearly state when you wish to *change the topic*, or to *introduce a new topic* for consideration.

- You should also state explicitly when you wish to cite another *example of the patient's behavior* that supports what another staff member has already cited. Or, if you wish to cite examples that seem to contradict the examples, or the conclusions, of other team members.

Weekend "Retreats" for the Staff. Once or twice a year, the staff should have a 2- to 3-day weekend "retreat." In these "retreats," theoretical issues and special clinical techniques should be discussed, debated, or role-played by the staff.

Self-Rating Documents. As part of the team training, members of the staff are also asked to perform self-ratings in several areas. These self-ratings are anonymous so that each person will have maximum incentive to self-disclose strengths and weaknesses without embarrassment. The group results are then shared with the staff and discussed further to explore what they imply in terms of "becoming first-class professionals in the field." Examples of two self-rating questionnaires follow.

Chapter 4 DVD, Vol 1, presents edited video clips that illustrate different types of team deliberations.

Table 4.1. Self-Rating Questionnaire 1

A. How am I viewed by my peers?

1. How do they feel about me personally?	They are "neutral" about me	I am liked by most	None like me	Some like me and some dislike me	All like me
2. How do my peers view my dedication?	Never viewed as really dedicated	Have some reservations about it	Always very dedicated	They are "neutral" about it	As fairly dedicated
3. Do they view me to be a "natural" team player?	Always, as a "natural" team player	Only as one who is trying to be a team player	They are "neutral" about it	Frequently a genuinely "natural" team player	Never viewed as a real "team player"
4. Do they respect my "professionalism"?	Never, really	They are "neutral" about it	With some reservations	With many reservations	Always, without reservations
5. Do they view me as an empathic and caring person?	With some reservations	With many reservations	As neither really a caring nor an empathic person	As only "average" in empathy	As an always caring and empathic person
6. How do they feel about my usual style as team deliberator?	Often have mixed feelings about it	"Neutral" about it	Always positive about it	On rare occasions they are impressed	Usually are annoyed by it
7. How do they rate my usual style of verbal communication?	Succinct and clear	Only fairly clear and succinct	Verbose as well as unclear	Verbose but clear	Succinct but unclear

B. How do I assess myself?

8. As a professional writer, I am:	Ineffective and need much editing	Below average; need much editing	Just fair; need only minor editing	Always effective; need no editing	Just fair; need much editing
9. As an analytical thinker, I am:	Occasionally a fair analyst	Often, adequate analytically	Always above average	On rare occasions, adequate analytically	Always weak in this area

(Continued)

Table 4.1. (*Contd.*)

B. How do I assess myself?

10. As a cognitive trainer (teacher) one on one, I am:	Mostly below average	Excellent	Fair in general	Fair but with some reservations	Mostly ineffective
11. As a personal and family counselor, I am:	Below average mostly; and need much supervision	Mostly average; need some supervision	Below average; need much more training and supervision	Above average mostly; need only minor supervision	Excellent; need no supervision
12. As group leader and "community" sessions leader, I am:	Weak in many ways	Average in both, without reservations	Generally below average in both	Average but with some reservations	Excellent in both

Table 4.2. Self-Rating Questionnaire 2

		Best rating				Worst rating
		5	4	3	2	1
Selflessness						
1.	My tendency is not to ask: "What's in it for me?" Rather, it is to consider the best interests of the trainees and the program.	5	4	3	2	1
2.	When necessary, I am willing/able to put in personal hours in my work, asking no remuneration.	5	4	3	2	1
Loyalty						
3.	I am loyal to my peers and supervisors.	5	4	3	2	1
Decision making						
4.	I am able to get to the "essentials" and to show decisiveness in work-related issues.	5	4	3	2	1

(Continued)

Table 4.2. (*Contd.*)

		Best rating				Worst rating
"Feel" or intuition						
5.	In dealing with clinical issues, I often rely on my intuition.	5	4	3	2	1
Aversion to "yes men"						
6.	I am capable of expressing reasoned disagreement.	5	4	3	2	1
7.	But, once a decision was arrived at, I am able to implement it even if initially I objected to it.	5	4	3	2	1
Informed, competent						
8.	I am knowledgeable about my field.	5	4	3	2	1
9.	I expect my peers and supervisors to be knowledgeable as well.	5	4	3	2	1
10.	I feel that I am competent as a therapeutic communicator.	5	4	3	2	1
11.	I feel that I have persuasive qualities (i.e., I can get across my ideas convincingly).	5	4	3	2	1
Mentorship						
12.	I like mentoring young professionals in my field and am good at it.	5	4	3	2	1
Consideration						
13.	I am considerate of my peers'/ subordinates' well-being.	5	4	3	2	1
14.	I am good at sponsoring and aiding the advancement of younger and less experienced psychologists.	5	4	3	2	1

(Continued)

Table 4.2. (*Contd.*)

		Best rating				Worst rating
Delegating responsibilities						
15.	I can delegate responsibility and authority to others who are supervised by me.	5	4	3	2	1
16.	I value originality and independence in others and expect quality results from their work.	5	4	3	2	1
17.	I can be counted on to "deliver" on my assignments.	5	4	3	2	1
Problem solver						
18.	I am a good problem solver.	5	4	3	2	1
19.	I am not a "fixer." Rather, I prefer pointing out how things could be handled.	5	4	3	2	1
Analysis						
20.	I prefer that all sides of an issue be considered and thoroughly debated.	5	4	3	2	1

Evaluating the Program Director as Clinical Leader

To paraphrase the famous saying, "Beauty is in the eye of the beholder," the program director and chief clinician should also exhibit, by his or her overall attitude and actual behaviors, the qualities of moral courage, openness, and willingness to explore and self-examine how the members of the team view him or her.

To obtain the truest "picture" of how members of the staff perceived and felt about him or her as a professional and as a leader, staff members were asked (for example) to respond (in a typed format and anonymously) to the following questions:

1. Which of [YBY's] personality and leadership qualities do you appreciate?

2. Which of these qualities would you personally wish to emulate?

3. Which of his personality qualities, or aspects of his style of communication, or his behavior, annoy you most or frustrate you?

Results of this anonymous "survey" were quite informative and provided the author with much food for thought. The following direct quotations (bracketed comments are the author's) are illustrative:

Concerning the first question (qualities most appreciated):

- "[His] enthusiasm and energy… are endless. He is always working [or] methodically plotting out an approach to treatment… [his] creativity when considering ways [how] to approach complex clinical issues."

- "[His] incredible charisma."

- "[His] team- focus and humility. For example, he does not need to take credit for his ideas on how to work with patients or their significant others. [He] will always suggest that the staff member take credit for ideas that [were] really his."

- "[The way] he [lets] junior members of the staff speak first, before he gives his opinion."

- "His interest in teaching members of the staff as well as his openness to visiting professionals."

- "[The way he] doesn't let red tape influence his clinical decisions. This shows [that] he is more concerned with the welfare of the patient [rather] than making a profit."

- "[The way] he treats everyone equally… [the way he wants] everyone [to] contribute in decision making."

- "[His] pragmatic, deliberate, and creative problem-solving style."

- "[The way he] has a story appropriate for every situation [which] has a humanizing and simplifying effect on the most perplexing clinical issues."

- "His dedication; intelligence; creativity; positive outlook; and decisiveness."

- "[He] is a 'player-coach.' He rolls up his 'sleeves' and participates in the program on all levels."

- "His passion about his field and [the willingness] to share his knowledge and experience... his enthusiasm."

Concerning qualities or behaviors that annoyed or frustrated:

- "[He] can be impatient [and make] harsh criticisms which ultimately [tend to lead] to constriction in group deliberations."

- "... he sometimes puts people on the spot [which] embarrasses them."

- "[Working] with such a person can be... anxiety provoking [because] one is expected to be on the mark—always. [However] although difficult, at times, it comes with the territory of learning from the best."

- "Sometimes [he] sends mixed messages within the same statement."

- "[He can be at times] overbearing [when he is displeased with the way the] staff communicates... However, this is understandable because, in this field, the bar for clear communication should be set high."

- "[His] impatience, irritability and [blunt] style of communication [are often] humiliating or embarrassing [when done in the presence of other staff]."

- "[His manner of] challenging [people] to think harder intimidates and causes people to shut down and [to be] unable to think clearly."

Table 4.3. A Staff Candidate's Personal and Professional Attributes Under Scrutiny

	Area	Specific characteristics/aspects
I	Body language definition: Does the candidate exhibit the "body language"—the demeanor, tone of voice, and poise—to suggest that he or she:	(a) Can control the anxiety or discomfort that a person experiences when being observed and interviewed by a group of interviewers while being somewhat physically "isolated" from the group and a video camera is recording the proceedings? (b) Can think and calmly respond to probing (but never hostile) questions? (c) Can give reasonably coherent answers?
II	Knowledge base	(a) Is the candidate familiar with neuropsychological concepts? (b) Is the candidate familiar with the typical behavioral manifestations of neurological impairments of cognitive or affective functions? (c) Is the candidate familiar with the types of behaviors that are manifested by non-brain-injured persons who have different types of adjustment problems?
III	Observing and interpreting facts or situations	(a) How good is the candidate in observing and interpreting his or her personal experiences in the here and now? (b) How good is the candidate in drawing inferences from what interviewers say during the interview? (c) Does the candidate tend to evaluate the meaning of observations based on his or her phenomenological experience or in terms of some theoretical formulations in books?
IV	Style of arriving at conclusions	(a) Does the candidate exhibit, primarily, an inductive or deductive reasoning style? (b) Does the candidate exhibit the ability to question or alter his or her conclusions if presented with new facts that tend to contradict his or her initial conclusion?

(Continued)

Table 4.3. (*Contd.*)

	Area	Specific characteristics/aspects
V	Style of verbal communication	(a) Does the candidate exhibit a verbose style of communicating thoughts, or a tendency to be succinct while answering questions?
		(b) Does the candidate tend to use jargon or stereotypical expressions, or to speak by using "plain" language?
		(c) If challenged by an unexpected question, does the candidate tend to admit to not having an immediate answer to the question, or will the candidate tend to "filibuster" (i.e., launch into long "speeches" in an obvious attempt to "buy time")?
VI	The candidate's perception of self as a "helper"	(a) Does the candidate perceive himself or herself as an inspirational (or "charismatic") type when acting as a "helper," or, does he or she view himself or herself as being a teacher, or, therapist/"coach" when attempting to correct the errors of a patient?
		(b) If the candidate sees himself or herself to be a "little bit of all three," does the candidate have an idea (or can he or she estimate) what proportion of the three helping types characterize his or her style?
VII	Self-knowledge and the "courage" to self-disclose	(a) Is the candidate aware of his or her "strong" (or attractive) personality characteristics, and is he or she willing, i.e., have the "courage" to, admit to some of his or her weaknesses as well?
VIII	Flexibility	(a) Does the candidate exhibit, in behavior and words, flexibility—i.e., adaptability—in new situations?
IX	Stamina	(a) Does the candidate appear to be a high-energy type of person, i.e., who possesses the stamina needed for long working hours?
X	Accepting and benefiting from constructive criticisms	(a) Does the candidate see himself or herself as a person who can "absorb" constructive criticism, without becoming emotionally "bruised" too much by it?

Selecting New Staff Candidates

Years of experience have shown that for a complex and demanding holistic program, such as ours, the best way of assembling a suitable staff is to recruit postdoctoral fellows and train them "on the job" for a year or two. The following "recruitment" procedure has been adopted:

1. A new applicant is interviewed jointly by all members of the staff.

2. The candidate is seated in a somewhat "isolated" spot from the rest of the staff, and a video camera is set up so that the proceedings can be recorded. The candidate is informed that a copy of the videotaped interview will be provided to him or her.

3. At the end of the interview, all members of the staff provide honest but tactfully delivered feedback to the candidate.

4. Since neither the academic education nor the clinical training (prior to the candidate's application) prepares the individual for what he or she is expected to experience in this "therapeutic community" setting, it does not make much sense to inquire in depth about previous experiences the candidate may have had in other settings. Thus, the interview is focused on assessing the candidate's temperamental and personality characteristics as well as whether or not he or she possesses the necessary clinical skills (or the potential for developing such skills). Hence, the areas that are focused on during the interviews are outlined below.

DVD Illustrations

Volume 1 provides edited video clips from a group interview of a new staff candidate.

Volume 2 presents edited video clips that illustrate different types of team deliberations.

Chapter 5 | *Identifying and Assessing Potential Program Trainees*

This chapter (1) describes the procedure for identifying potential candidates for the program, (2) outlines the specific areas that are the focus of the assessment of new candidates, and (3) presents two clinical case studies. These six cases are a representative sample of the types of patients who were typically evaluated in our setting; enrolled into our program; and, ultimately, have benefitted from it. The first case ("Laura") typifies individuals who seek acceptance into the program voluntarily. The second case ("Brendan") illustrates those individuals who initially were recalcitrant, but who, in time, "converted" to becoming voluntary program trainees as well. And the third case ("Martha"), the fourth case ("Raquel,") the fifth case ("Jack"), and the sixth case ("Liz") respectively, typify a subset of brain-injured individuals—who can be described as "problematic" patients. Such problematic patients, enrolled into our program, participated, initially only half-heartedly, or prior to entering our program they had rejected neuropsychological rehabilitation altogether. But, gradually they have become genuinely committed both to the philosophy of our program, as well as to practicing the various cognitive-remedial and therapeutic "exercises" that are being offered in our setting.

To provide a background against which these cases studies should be evaluated, we briefly reiterate the order in which eight overlapping (interim) clinical objectives, or "landmarks," are being pursued by our program. Accordingly, the first objective is to obtain the patient's voluntary consent to enter our program. The second objective is to help the patient become aware of and understand the nature of the cognitive deficits, the neurobehavioral impairments, and the functional consequences of his or her brain injury. The third objective is to ameliorate problems with impulse control, or problems with the initiation of (and the ability to sustain) purposeful behaviours (such as engaging in learning or training experiences. The fourth clinical objective is to ameliorate problems in attention and concentration, so that the patient can become an effective student (i.e., capable of achieving optimal results during the four stages that will follow). Thus, during the fifth, sixth, seventh, and eight clinical "landmarks," respectively, the objectives are to: improve the speed and the efficiency of information processing; ameliorate the effects of the memory disorders; help the patient to learn compensatory skills (to be capable of enhancing his or her functional competencies); and help the patient to regain a positive sense of self (or "ego-identity"), which will make it possible for the patient to find meaning in his or her achievements following rehabilitation.

Identifying Potential Candidates

Invitation to Observe the Program

Whenever practically possible, a candidate is invited to visit the program, accompanied by significant others, to observe (free of charge) the program for 1 to 2 days. In addition to providing the new candidate the opportunity to observe the program and the way trainees and their significant others are treated by the staff, such visits also enable the staff to observe how the candidate interacts with the other trainees, and how both the candidate and his or her significant other interact with the program staff. If all goes well, a date is set for a formal assessment.

The Assessment

The initial assessment takes place typically between 3 and 5 consecutive days. It consists of:

- A clinical interview;

- Procedures to estimate the candidate's preinjury intellectual aptitude (or IQ range);

■ Administration of a comprehensive battery of neuropsychological and cognitive tests, designed to assess the current integrity of basic neuropsychological functions (e.g., the presence or the absence, and the extent of severity, of frontal-lobe disinhibition and/or adynamic symptoms; attention and concentration functions; speed and efficiency of cognitive functions; memory functions and learning abilities) and the candidate's cognitive abilities (e.g., visuoperceptual integrative and information-processing skills, language and communication skills; and higher level reasoning abilities);

■ Procedures designed to assess the validity of the candidate's test results (i.e., whether the test findings may be considered to be an accurate reflection of the candidate's current true abilities);

■ Remedial probes designed to assess the candidate's potential to benefit from systematic (individualized and group) cognitive training procedures, and whether or not the candidate would prove able to respond to individualized and group psychotherapeutic interventions, specially modified to suit the needs of brain-injured individuals);

■ Procedures aimed at assessing the presence in the candidate's personality of those characteristics that will enable him or her to ultimately attain an optimal postrehabilitative functional adjustment.

The Clinical Interview

The clinical interview is aimed at obtaining answers to questions such as:

■ Is the candidate sufficiently alert, attentive, and capable of engaging in the give-and-take of a clinical interview?

■ Is the candidate aware of (and able to admit) that the injury has affected his or her functional life, to the point where preinjury work-study goals may not be possible to attain (without modifications)?

- Can the candidate cite some specific functions that have been affected by the injury?

- Is the candidate aware of the possibility that deficits that have resulted from the injury will not "go away" with time and rest (like a flu, for example)?

- Is the candidate willing to consider the possibility that he or she may require specialized rehabilitative interventions (as opposed to receiving "tutorial help in math," for example)?

- If specialized rehabilitation is recommended, will the candidate be able to accept such help by trusting the professionals, even if, initially, he or she may not understand the rationale for such interventions?

- Can the candidate cite some example, from his or her preinjury past, when systematic training by trusted "coaches" has resulted in the improvement of some of his or her skills?

- How good is the candidate as an observer of facts or the behaviors of others?

- How well is the candidate able to identify some of his or her core personality characteristics, and how capable is the candidate of identifying the same in his or her significant others, friends, or strangers whom he or she has just met?

- Does the candidate possess the ability to react to humorous comments?

- Does the candidate behave in a socially appropriate manner in one-on-one or group situations?

Acceptance into the program is, thus, based on the outcomes of all the assessment procedures.

Case Study 1: ("Laura")

Laura was a 52-year-old divorced woman with two grown sons from her previous marriage. Prior to her two consecutive motor vehicle accidents (both as a pedestrian), she was a high-powered marketing executive and creative director at a world-renowned publishing house. A Yale University graduate, she was described as having had "superb" organizational skills, capacity for logical-analytic reasoning, and managerial skills. Letters from former colleagues and employers contained characterizations such as: "extremely logical, creative, and intelligent, accustomed to taking charge and handling a lot of responsibility both personally and professionally"; "highly visual, organized, persistent, decisive, and articulate"; "communicated well on paper and verbally"; "a problem solver, quick to analyze a situation, grasp the problem and able to formulate solutions quickly, no matter how complex"; "able to see things [intellectually and visually] from more than one angle at once."

After divorcing her husband, Laura fell into a depression and was diagnosed as bipolar. She would initially become manic and then depressed. Reportedly, she spent a good year struggling to get the depression under control, and not too long after she did so, she was hit by a car while crossing the street. This was her first accident.

Laura's depression, reportedly, started "6 months after I left my husband of 23 years (although I was prone to it my entire life). It was quite severe for a while. I was put on a series of antidepressants (with psychotherapy) continuing to the present."

After her first accident, she was out of work for 2 weeks (while recovering from the accident); after which, she resumed working. But she resigned from the company where she worked for 7 years and started the process of creating a business as a freelance consultant. However, in her new enterprise, she was able to do part-time work for only a few weeks, when the second accident occurred. This time, she was hit by a motorcycle while crossing the street against a traffic light. Following the second accident, she was no longer able to work again.

In her first accident, Laura claimed that her head had "cracked the windshield" of the car. But she experienced no loss of consciousness at this time and was hospitalized for two nights only. Reportedly, she sustained no other injuries "other than bruising and a mild concussion." She described herself after her first accident in this way: "I became overwhelmed [when] working on my own and found it hard to proceed with projects I wanted to create. Each step was difficult, even making appointments with people, despite my excellent standing in the industry and [excellent] personal relationships." Her difficulties at the time, were described as

- *"Hard to get motivated [i.e., to] self-start."*

- *"Friends noticed incidents of memory loss... and thought that this wasn't like me" (i.e., that memory lapses were not typical of her, as they knew her).*

- *"Family members noticed that I sometimes acted spaced out and sometimes was slower in my reactions"*

Following her second accident, Laura reportedly had severely impaired "short-term memory"; "woke up confused and didn't remember much about the previous day"; "spoke to my family clearly one minute, then said things that made no sense"; and was not "completely lucid," though she persisted in acting in her customary "take-charge" manner.

Laura further reported that, after her second accident, she had "trouble with coordination of fine motor skills" (dropping things, clumsiness, and weakened hands).

As to her cognitive functions, Laura cited (during her interview with her examiner at our program) several persisting problems:

- *She could recall only "occasional events" from her hospital stay.*

- *She reported that short-term memory problems were "still very difficult" to take.*

- *She could not recall having spoken "multiple times" with friends, yet she thought that they "had not known about" her accident.*

- *She "mixed up," at times, the chronology of events.*

- *Her "thought processes" were "muddled and disoriented at times."*

- *She had "trouble following long stories or remembering where they started and where they were going."*

- *While writing, she found that her thoughts would "meander." Periodically she experienced difficulties "finding words." Or, that she tended to "lose [her] train of thought."*

- *She found it hard "to take answers to their next step in understanding."*

- *She was "unable to deduct the big picture" or even "ask [on the spot] for further clarification."*

- *Her brain, in general, was not "as nimble as before the accident" and she felt that she "cannot handle layered [i.e., multimeaning] ideas."*

- *While reading, her "concentration and retention [were] not up to [her] previous levels."*

- *Her attention span was "shortened."*

- *She committed "absent-minded" behaviors, such as "attempting to drink from an empty glass," or trying to "pour a bottle with the lid on."*

- *Generally, she felt that her brain was "overloaded and overwhelmed at times."*

Test-Taking Attitude and Clinical Observations. *Laura was cooperative throughout and eager to respond to all the examiner's requests. She openly conveyed her self-observations and (quite obviously) made consistent efforts to perform tests as best as she could.*

She routinely, and audibly, engaged her verbal skills while performing nonverbal tests that required planning or sequential execution. She commented frequently (while performing a computerized hierarchy of tests of basic attention and concentration) that she was "so focused on anticipating the onset of the signal ['go'] light" that she could not "see the number on the screen" (i.e., her attention was so hyperfocused on the signal light that she missed "seeing the screen," which indicated the speed of her reaction time).

When provided with verbal instructions or explanations, Laura repeatedly said: "I don't understand what you are saying." The examiner reliably ascertained that the problem was not due to receptive aphasia but rather to a decrease in the time efficiency of her information processing (i.e., she clearly remembered what she was told but needed more time to comprehend).

While she performed (quite accurately) an untimed visual test, which called for the detection of subtle similarities and differences between different visual shapes, she burst into tears and cried out: "I can't stand this, it is so hard!" As she explained, such tasks were part of her work before. But she quickly recovered her "businesslike" and calm demeanor, ready to proceed with the testing.

Laura's test findings were summarized, under separate headings, as follows:

Basic Attentional Functions. *On a computerized test hierarchy that assessed the current integrity of three components of her basic attention and concentration—vigilance, the ability to discriminate between different visual stimuli, and the ability to concentrate (i.e., track a train of thought while screening out irrelevant internal or external stimuli)—she was found to be impaired on all three aspects of her basic attentional functions.*

Eye–Hand Coordination with Finger Dexterity. *Laura scored with her right (dominant) hand at the 4th percentile, compared with female college students, and only at the 2nd percentile level when she performed a peg-placing test. She was clearly impaired on this standard dexterity measure, thus confirming her own subjective observations concerning her diminished dexterity following her injuries.*

Visual-Perceptual-Spatial Integrative Functions. *An array of visual information processing tests revealed that*

- *Laura's time-efficiency was (abnormally) slowed. But the accuracy of her linear visual scanning and cancellation was found to be normal.*

- *Likewise, she performed normally on tests that involved dynamic visual scanning and the need to detect subtle similarities and differences among familiar or unfamiliar figures.*

- *However, Laura performed within the borderline–normal range on a series of tests involving visual pattern analysis.*

- *Also normal were her performances on various constructional praxis tests.*

All in all, in this domain, her functioning was found to remain essentially within normal limits.

Language and Communication Skills. *Laura was found to be moderately impaired on a test that requires mental control and the ability to generate words beginning with the same letter. However, on tests of verbal comprehension, she was found to be normal when compared to people with her level of intelligence, education, and sophistication.*

Laura's ability to express her thoughts in writing was also found to be normal (i.e., commensurate with her preinjury abilities).

Learning and Memory Functions. *Laura's memory functions were found to be within the normal limits on some tests, within the borderline range on some of the tests, and impaired, to various degrees, on yet other tests. The formal test results confirmed her own and her family and friend's observations concerning her memory lapses. It is noteworthy that her greatest vulnerabilities, in the memory domain, were revealed to be on tests that were verbally based, but less so on visually based tests.*

Higher Level Reasoning Functions. *Although Laura obtained scores within the superior intellectual range on a general intellectual aptitude test (WAIS-III) IQ, both on the verbal as well as the performance scales, Laura's performances on special tests that were designed to assess the integrity of the three aspects of her higher level reasoning functions—(a) her convergent reasoning abilities, (b) her divergent reasoning abilities, and (c) her "executive" functions—fluctuated between the normal and the moderately impaired ranges. Thus, her performances on such tests revealed an unreliability of her higher level reasoning abilities, due to either her emotional states or the inadequacy of her attention and concentration, or both.*

Results of Remedial Probes. *To assess whether Laura was a good candidate for our program, she underwent two remedial probes as follows:*

1. Testing her potential to benefit from systematic cognitive remedial interventions. When she was initially tested, Laura was found to be impaired on three reaction time paradigms, which measure the integrity of the vigilance and self-induction component of her basic attentional functions. The remedial probe consisted of 100 trials during which special auditory cues were designed to facilitate her vigilance, the formation of an anticipatory mental set (e.g., expecting the onset of the stimulus "go" light after the warning "get set"), or her self-induction (i.e., the mental preparation needed to react as fast as she could when the signal light came on). The cues were systematically and gradually reduced from maximum cues through variations of partial cues, to no cues at all.

Upon completion of the remedial training session (for about 2 hours), Laura was retested on the three computerized reaction time tests to see if (a) she succeeded in establishing a "learning curve" and (b) whether as a result of the remedial training a "transfer of learning" took place. Results are summarized in Table 5.1.

As can be seen, Laura proved able to benefit from systematic remedial training and was, thus, deemed to be an excellent candidate for our program.

2. Ability to benefit from small-group psychotherapeutic interventions in a "therapeutic community" setting. In the presence of a peer group, their significant others, and the entire staff, Laura was interviewed by the examiner and had the opportunity to interact with the other trainees. The purpose of this group interview was to assess whether

- She was willing and able to engage in such group sessions.

- She possessed the minimum empathic abilities needed for establishing rapport with peers.

Table 5.1. Results of Remedial Probe in the Attentional Domain

Tests	Score at baseline	Score after the probe
1. Visual reaction time		
(a) Variable intervals	331 ms Mildly impaired	228 ms Normal
(b) Constant intervals	328 ms Mildly impaired	215 ms Normal
2. Attention Reaction Conditioner, ARC	6.0 lights Moderately impaired	7.5 lights Normal

- *She was capable of being inspired by her peers and, in turn, of inspiring her peers in their struggle to overcome their problems.*

- *She would be willing to accept "coaching" and constructive criticisms.*

Laura revealed herself to be a warm, empathic, and "egalitarian" person with excellent "people skills." She received uniformly excellent feedback from all the participants. They all felt that she would be a welcome member of this "therapeutic community" and "predicted" that she would benefit greatly if she were to enroll into the program.

Laura promptly enrolled into our program and, after a few weeks, actually commenced her treatments.

Outcome

After "graduating" from the program, Laura was asked to become a "peer counselor." She performed with distinction having become a role model for successful rehabilitation to her peers as well as their significant others. Then, some time afterward, Laura enrolled into graduate studies, at a Washington, D.C. university, where (as of this writing) she has been pursuing (academic) studies toward becoming a rehabilitation counselor.

Case Study 2 ("Brendan")

At the age of 20, Brendan, a handsome, tall, and athletic young man, was brought to New York by his mother, hoping that he would agree to join our program. Brendan suffered a traumatic brain injury 3 years earlier as a result of a motor vehicle accident on a cold winter day in Texas.

The accident occurred when Brendan, who was driving a car that belonged to his mother's business, slipped on the icy road, spun around, and hit a concrete wall. Brendan was not wearing his seat belt. He was thrown out of the car and lost consciousness at the scene of the accident. He was found by the police and was admitted at the local medical center with multiple traumas, including head injuries.

A cranial CT scan revealed multiple hemorrhagic contusions in the cortex and the subcortical white matter of his left frontal lobe. His third ventricle was compressed. Brendan was also diagnosed as having a subarachnoid hemorrhage, a small subdural hematoma, and a basilar skull fracture. X-rays further revealed the presence of fractures in his wrist and multiple left rib fractures.

A phenobarbital coma was induced, and he underwent hyperventilation with Manitol to control intracranial pressure. Brendan developed right lower-lobe pneumonia and penicillin-resistant staph infection. He also developed a body rash, as a reaction to Dilantin. Subsequently, he experienced painful neuropathy involving his lower extremities and was treated with ivy morphine. Brendan was in a comatose state for approximately three and a half weeks.

Brenda's mother was a 49-year-old divorced woman who raised her three children (Bredan was the middle son) as a single parent. She was an astute businesswoman who managed several successful businesses.

Reportedly, Brendan was never a good student because he was diagnosed as having been dyslexic since the second grade. Brendan "hated" all the academic studies at school. But he was a "star" athlete and was very popular with the girls. At the age of 17, Brendan decided to quit school and go to work for his mother in one of her businesses.

However, after a while, he obtained a GED (a certificate that he graduated from high school) following intensive tutorials. Brendan felt that obtaining a GED was important since he planned to some day take over his mother's businesses. While he was still a high school student, Brendan's math skills were above average, and despite being a poor student in all the verbal-based subjects, he was considered by his teachers to be an intelligent and "charming" young man.

Upon regaining consciousness, Brendan was transferred to Baylor Institute for Rehabilitation (a renowned institute in Texas). At Baylor, he was treated with Coumadin for possible pulmonary embolism and underwent various rehabilitative therapies. He also evidenced mild, flaccid dysarthria and aphasia (predominantly word-finding difficulties), which improved significantly with speech therapy.

Brendan was discharged from Baylor (after 3 months of intensive rehabilitation) and sent to another center for follow-up physical and speech therapies. Brendan steadfastly denied that he needed further rehabilitation *and refused to attend the nearby outpatient program. In addition, his adjustment was problematic due to his impulsive behavior, frequent and extreme temper flare-ups, seizures, and poor judgment. (At the time, Brendan was on Neuroutin—400 mg × 3—to prevent seizures.) During the 3 years between his injury and his assessment at our facility, Brendan underwent several neuropsychological evaluations. These evaluations revealed that superimposed on his long-standing problems with "dyslexia" and academic difficulties were many "new" neurobehavioral and cognitive impairments that resulted from the brain injury sustained in the motor vehicle accident.*

Brendan's mother was very much stressed by her son's behavior and worried a great deal about his future. Brendan himself was unhappy about the situation because he was very fond of his mother and realized that his erratic behavior caused her much pain.

After his mother's pleadings, Brendan agreed to come to New York to "take a look" at our program. But, immediately upon his arrival, he declared that he came "only to please" his mother and that he did not feel that he needed rehabilitation. While he agreed to undergo testing, he repeatedly stated that he was dyslexic and that he hated taking "any kind of tests." He consented to have his mother sit in and observe while he was being tested (in fact, he invited her to do so).

Upon hearing Brendan's "declaration" that he agreed to come to New York "just to please" his mother, the examiner addressed the mother (while, actually, with "paradoxical intention," the examiner's aim was to be heard by Brendan):

> *Mrs. _W._____, you are, in my opinion, a very fortunate lady for having such a loving son. Even though he does not think that he needs rehabilitation, he came to New York, just to please you. But, I must tell you frankly: If by the end of this evaluation period, your son will remain still unconvinced that he needs rehabilitation, we will recommend that you take him back home to Texas. Because we do not "take prisoners" into this program. Only volunteers. Our experience over the years has been that people who agreed to join our program just because they loved their mother did not benefit at all. So, if after a few days Brendan will still say, "I don't need rehabilitation(!)," you should take him back to Texas.*

Although Brendan said nothing, it was quite clear that he was "impressed" by the examiner's comments to his mother. His somewhat surly behavior, up to that point, gave way to a cooperative, even friendly, attitude afterward. And so, over the next 5 days, Brendan observed different treatment sessions in our program, socialized with our trainees and their significant others, and underwent comprehensive testing.

On the fourth day, Brendan and his mother received an oral summary of the highlights of the findings (an extensive written report was to follow). The examiner, being mindful of Brendan's long-standing negative feelings about receiving "bad news" concerning his academic difficulties, made it a special point to report, first, some "good news." Addressing both Brendan and his mother, the examiner told them that he found "some very pleasant surprises" upon analyzing the test results, such as

▪ *"On 12 computerized tests of attention and concentration, you performed in a perfectly normal way. This is encouraging because it shows that you have a potential to benefit from cognitive training."*

▪ *"You were also found to be accurate, and fairly fast, in detecting similarities and differences among visual shapes. These test results show that the visual area is your greatest asset, and since you remain quite able to coordinate your two hands, while performing some hands-on, practical tasks (which explains why you were such a good athlete...!), you'll have a good chance to become a productive worker again in the future."*

▪ *"But on many tests that involve answering questions verbally or in writing, the results—as we might expect—show that your accident has weakened those skills, even more than they were before your accident."*

While Brendan accepted the "good news" with apparent equanimity, upon hearing the examiner's comment that his brain injuries had exacerbated his previous deficits in the verbal-ideational domains, he became hostile, agitated, and verbally abusive. Using many vulgar expressions, he accused the examiner of being "just like the others" (meaning like the other psychologists in Texas). Again, he reiterated, "I didn't come here to hear all this [expletive]." Brendan's mother was obviously mortified by her son's outburst. But the examiner, who throughout Brendan's outburst remained silent and assumed a calm demeanor, addressed the mother in a soft and empathic tone (once again, his comments were intended for Brendan's ears as well):

> *Mrs.__W.____, please don't be upset. Although I don't agree with Brendan, I understand why he feels this way. You see, for many years, before his accident, he always knew that he was a smart guy. He loved you and wanted you to feel proud of him. But his dyslexia made it impossible for him to be a smart student academically. Only by being an excellent athlete was he able to make you feel proud of him. In his gut, however, he became "allergic" to being tested all the time and receiving bad news. He developed a dislike for such examiners because, to him, it must have felt that they thought he was either "stupid" or "unmotivated." But he must have felt that his dedicated and disciplined behavior toward his sport coaches should have told them that they were wrong. So, I don't blame Brendan for letting me have it. Even though, by telling him the truth, I showed him real respect!*

The examiner then reiterated what he said several days before that: "If Brendan will feel tomorrow the same way as he feels today, he will probably go home with you to Texas."

Case Study 3: "Martha"

At the age of 24, Martha enrolled into our program. Four years earlier—at the age of 19—Martha was a high-achieving college student and a star athlete. After attending a collegiate sport competition event, Martha was involved in a major motor vehicle accident.

Background

Martha is the eldest of three siblings. Her father, an alcoholic, has been divorced from her mother many years prior to the accident. Her mother, an attractive, nondrinker and competent single parent, managed the secretarial staff of a large business office. Martha has a close and loving relationship with her mother.

Both of Martha's younger siblings were abusing drugs and were academically low achievers. On the other hand, Martha, who never drank or used drugs, excelled academically and in sports and helped her mother in managing the household chores. After graduating from high school, at the top of her class, Martha received a full scholarship from an elite college.

Consequences of the Motor Vehicle Accident

Acute Hospitalization. *During the motor vehicle accident, Martha sustained left ventricular hemorrhage and frontal and parietooccipital contusions. She was comatose for 9 days, and her posttraumatic amnesia (PTA) was reported to have lasted for 14 days. Upon emerging from the PTA, she was described as having had multiple cognitive impairments, a mild left hemiparesis, and depression.*

Postacute Rehabilitation. *After she was discharged from acute (inpatient) hospitalization, Martha was enrolled in two outpatient rehabilitation programs in her city. But she was described as "uncooperative" and as a person who "could not be reached and persuaded to accept the consequences of her injury." After some weeks, Martha discharged herself, against medical advice, and decided to work hard, on her own, toward returning to her college studies. Martha was unwilling to accept the idea that rehabilitation could not "guarantee" her full recovery and the ability to resume her previous academic studies.*

Failure to Self-Rehabilitate. *Having discharged herself from both rehabilitation programs, Martha spent many hours at the local library and began to work part-time as a "check-out" person at a local supermarket. But she failed repeatedly at both tasks. Her depression became worse and her personal and social isolation even more pronounced than before.*

Martha Is Persuaded by Her Mother to Enroll in Our Program. *Nearly 4 years after her injury, at her mother's urging, Martha agreed to enter our program. Her decision was based on her mother's promise to also participate in our program to the extent that her job would permit. (The owner of the mother's company reassured her that she would be permitted to take time off from work from time to time.) On our initial neuropsychological evaluation of Martha, we found her to be a highly intelligent and completely demoralized young woman who exhibited*

- ■ *Signs of frontal-lobe dysfunctioning, characterized by mild impulsiveness, difficulty to modulate (i.e., adjust or regulate) the expression of negative emotions, organic irritability and the tendency to ruminate (i.e., to obsessively be preoccupied with thoughts about things that irritated her)*

- *Problems with concentration because of a difficulty to "screen out" internal distracters*

- *Slowed-down speed and efficiency of information processing with subtle aphasic problems*

- *"Noisy listening"—a tendency to misunderstand or misinterpret what she was told (even while seemingly listening when spoken to, probably due to her internal preoccupation with her "private" interpretations of what she was told)*

- *Circumscribed (i.e., limited to some tests only) impairments of her memory functions*

- *Mild impairments of her higher level reasoning functions*

- *Pronounced self-critical and self-deprecatory behaviors when her test performances were less than "perfect" (as she saw it)*

- *A tendency to be withdrawn and socially uncomfortable in her interactions with peers or our staff.*

Martha's Gradual Positive Response to the Program Interventions. *Over a period of slightly longer than one year (i.e., over two cycles), Martha gradually "opened up", developed trust toward our staff and some of her peers, invested herself fully in the various individualized and group cognitive and therapeutic activities, and became a committed member of our therapeutic community. Although she experienced many tearful moments throughout, Martha revealed the hard-working tendencies, the dedication, and the persistence of the high-achieving academic student and star athlete that she was prior to her injury.*

As we gained insight into Martha's personality, we understood both her constant drive for excellence in all areas of her life, as well as her reason for rejecting rehabilitation before entering our program: Her constant drive to excel was, in part at least, motivated by her (largely unconscious) psychological defense against becoming addicted (to alcohol or drugs) like her father and siblings. Her rejection of rehabilitation and discharging herself against medical advice were in response to the constant "preaching" (as she perceived it) of the professionals that she "had to accept" her limitations. She felt that such "preaching" was a "message of surrender," a demand that she "become a pitiful cripple and second-rate human being."

Outcomes

After graduating from (two cycles of) intensive remedial and therapeutic interventions, Martha underwent part-time work trials at our medical center, where she performed clerical tasks, enrolled into a special college program to test out her ability to resume academic studies, and received personal counseling (often in joint sessions with her mother) during a third cycle.

Having achieved excellent results in all of the three foregoing areas, Martha secured a part-time paid clerical job, while pursuing a full-time academic program to become a qualified librarian. Two years later, she graduated cum laude and began working as a librarian at a college in her state.

Ten years after her injury, Martha married an airline pilot, became the mother of a bright and energetic little boy, and continues to work as a librarian.

Chapter 4 DVD, Volume 1 presents edited excerpts video clips of Martha's progress over a period of one and a half years.

Case Study 4: "Raquel"

At the time when Raquel enrolled into our program, she was 21 years old. She was one of two bright, high-achieving, high school students from the Philippine Islands who received a full-time scholarship from a well-known ("Ivy League") university in the United States, where she began to study psychology. One day, while walking to classes on her campus, Raquel was struck by a Federal Express truck. She was comatose for 3 weeks; sustained a skull fracture and right temporal contusions; suffered an initial seizure; sustained fractures to her right leg, pubic bones, left ribs, and collar bone; and had a left cranial nerve palsy.

Upon emerging from a coma, Raquel had no memory of the accident. She was hospitalized, as an inpatient, at a large rehabilitation center where she was treated for left hemiparesis, a left visual neglect, and multiple cognitive deficits. CT scans revealed the presence of subarachnoid hemorrhage, right temporal contusion, and a basilar skull fracture.

From the inpatient rehabilitation hospital, Raquel was transferred, for continued outpatient treatments, at another (well-known) rehabilitation center in New York. During her intake evaluation at the New York facility, Raquel exhibited mild deficits in her attention and concentration, moderate deficits in her memory functions, moderate impairments of her reasoning abilities (including deficiencies in problem solving), "impaired insight," mild auditory comprehension problems, difficulties in verbally expressing her thoughts, and some problems with the intelligibility of her speech.

But, the staff at the outpatient program found Raquel to be a particularly problematic patient. This was primarily because she steadfastly claimed to be "fine"; questioned the need for rehabilitation in her particular case; was stubborn, aggressive, and insulting in her interactions with her mother and the relatives with whom she and her mother resided in New York ("you don't understand anything"; "you should go for rehabilitation, not me"; "you lick the boots of the staff"). Because of her resistant and sullen (i.e., irritable, ill-humored) attitude, Raquel's mother had to beg her, daily, to go to the rehabilitation program and to cooperate. But she remained resistant.

As a last resort, Raquel was referred to our program. It was hoped that within the context of our therapeutic community a "breakthrough" might be achieved.

Findings from Our Initial Evaluation. *Over a period of 4 days (involving 18 hours of testing, interviews, and clinical observations), Raquel underwent an initial comprehensive assessment. Raquel was told that results of the evaluation "will be shared with you honestly" but that "we will not recommend that you enter our program unless you volunteer to enroll." Raquel was also told that "we insist that a candidate trainee voluntarily agree to enroll here and cooperate with our staff. We expect that the candidate agree to do so, even if our findings and explanations (concerning the rationale for the treatments) will not make sense at all." A summary of the key findings from our initial evaluation follows in the next few paragraphs.*

In the domain of basic attentional functions, Raquel exhibited moderate to severe impairments on tests of vigilance, self-induction, and reaction time; moderate to severe impairments on tests of discrimination between moving visual stimuli (but normal ability to discriminate between different stationary stimuli); and severe impairments on tests of concentration (i.e., tests that measured her ability to maintain a train of thought while effectively "screening out" irrelevant, distracter stimuli).

In the visual-perceptual-integrative functional domain, Raquel scored normally on tests involving linear visual scanning and cancellation, was moderately impaired on tests of dynamic visual scanning (i.e., identification of subtle similarities and differences among visual drawings), and scored within the moderately impaired range on tests involving analysis of complex visual patterns (which also called for logical reasoning).

In the domain of language and communications skills, Raquel scored within the mildly impaired range on a test that called for generating different words with the same first letter (a test of mental control), scored normally on a multiple-choice vocabulary test, but was moderately impaired on a multiple-choice test of reading comprehension. In written samples (measuring her ability to express her thoughts in writing), Raquel exhibited neither word-finding difficulties, nor grammatical nor syntactic errors (i.e., she exhibited no aphasic symptoms). But her reasoning ranged from idiosyncratic ways of viewing things to ways of reasoning that bordered on the illogical and expressed in ways (words) that one would not expect from a bright college student at an Ivy League university.

In the domain of her memory functions, Raquel scored differentially, with her scores ranging from (only) the borderline normal to the severely impaired range on verbal-based as well as visual-based tests of memory.

In the domain of her higher level reasoning, Raquel scored unevenly. Her scores ranged from the normal to the severely impaired range depending on the testing conditions. Thus, she scored differentially on tests that measured the intactness of her convergent thinking, divergent (and analytical) thinking, and her executive functions.

On a personality inventory, Raquel revealed the persistence of "old" (i.e., preinjury) tendencies, such as those to remain calm in times of stress; to be able to resist temptations (i.e., the ability to postpone pleasures); to value her privacy and to not show (outwardly) enthusiasm; a preference to stick to the tried and true; the tendency to engage in "logical" arguments; to be stubborn, skeptical, and guarded about disclosing her true feelings; and to dislike planning her activities in advance.

During one-on-one remedial probes in the cognitive area, Raquel showed that she could benefit from systematic training. But the carry-over effects of the remedial training were, clinically speaking, slow and only incremental. She did not appear to gain quick insights from her experiences. Nor was she able to draw logical inferences as would be expected from a college student on scholarship.

A small-group interview, designed to test Raquel's willingness and ability to participate in treatments with a peer group, revealed that she would, very likely, have difficulties empathizing with and trusting her peers and the staff. Nevertheless, Raquel agreed to voluntarily enter our program. (In our opinion, her agreement was based on her fear that if she admitted to having negative feelings about rehabilitation, she would be rejected by us.)

Overall Clinical "Picture" of Raquel at the End of the Intake Evaluation

On the basis of the clinical interviews (with Raquel and her mother), the test results, the remedial probes, and the many clinical observations (over several days), we concluded that Raquel

presented with a discontinuity, which was characterized by

■ A frontal lobe unawareness of the true nature and potential consequences of her deficits, and hence, her outright rejection of neuropsychological rehabilitation

■ An exacerbation, by her organic impairments of some of her preinjury personality characteristics (such as her skepticism, distrust of others, and her hypercritical tendencies). In combination, these represented significant alterations in Raquel's current personality. (Prior to her injury, she was described as polite, respectful toward her mother and other family members, and generally "obedient.")

■ Major impairments in her ability to correctly infer logical implications, from even her own accurate observations of facts. For example, Raquel correctly pointed out that her speed of reasoning became reduced by her injury, that she had difficulties "finding and using the right words to express [her] thoughts", and that her interpersonal relationships had deteriorated ("I am not the nice person I was before"). Yet, despite her being a psychology student and the foregoing accurate self-observations, she concluded that piano lessons,

*dance lessons, and math tutorials were what she needed. No wonder
our short- and long-term prognosis in Raquel's case was very
"guarded."*

Case Study 5: "Jack"

*About 4 years following a motor vehicle accident, at the age of 21, Jack
applied for entry into our program. Jack's history before entering our
program was very problematic in many respects, and our decision to accept
him into our program was made only after much hesitation.*

Jack's Injury

*Four years before Jack's application at our center, he was involved in a
motor vehicle accident. He was the driver of a car that rolled over after it
was hit by another car. It was reported that Jack had his seat belt fastened,
that he struck his head (possibly on the door), but that, apparently, he did
not lose consciousness. After he and the other passengers were extricated
from the car by the police, Jack said that he was "feeling all right." He was
taken to a nearby hospital but was released to his home on the same day.
However, 2 days later, Jack was examined by his pediatrician. His mother
complained that, since his accident, Jack was "forgetful," "easily distracted,"
"impulsive," "irritable," "moody," and "argumentative." The pediatrician
referred Jack for a neuropsychological evaluation, which commenced on the
following day.*

Summary of the First Neuropsychological Evaluation

*The clinical interviews (of Jack and his mother) by the neuropsychologist
revealed that Jack lived with his mother (an attorney), his father (an
accountant), and an older brother (who was away studying at college in a
different city) and that Jack was on Ritalin since he attended first grade
because he was diagnosed as having had an attentional disorder. However,
Jack was reported to have been "always smart, and academically advanced,
but socially immature" (i.e., that "he had problems getting along with other
children of his age"); in his second grade, Jack continued to perform very
well academically, but his social adjustment remained problematic. Then,
in high school his academic performance "fluctuated somewhat" and he had
to receive tutorial help twice a week. In his last year of high school (at the
age of 17), Jack sustained the "mild brain injuries" under discussion.*

Symptoms Manifested Following Jack's Accident

Jack complained of experiencing visual, auditory, and olfactory changes. He denied having headaches, balancing problems, or motor problems. His principal complaints were described, by various examiners, to include problems with memory and concentration, difficulties with word finding (but, as we interpreted these examiners' descriptions, the problem was dysarthria rather than aphasia), impulse control problems, and poor judgment (Jack himself described this by saying: "sometimes my judgment is off"). His mother noted that Jack began associating with individuals younger than himself and clearly implied that she and her husband found Jack's new friends undesirable. Jack acknowledged that while he was "feeling better," he was sad, had mood swings, and suffered from insomnia. He denied feelings of hopelessness or suicidal ideation. Jack's manner in his interactions with the psychologist was described as "reserved and casual."

Cognitive and Behavioral Findings. *The psychologist summarized the results of extensive testing and clinical observations. They revealed*

- *Mild cognitive residua of his accident*

- *Word-finding difficulties*

- *Problems with concentration*

- *Slowed speed of mental processing*

- *Some anxiety with concerns about the future (i.e., a fear that he may not be able to attain his preinjury ambitions)*

The first psychologist's recommendation was that, since Jack exhibited no "acute significant emotional distress," and since he was academically doing fairly well, only the psychopharmacological intervention (Ritalin) should be continued. But, the psychologist pointed out that should Jack's anxiety increase, "individual psychotherapy may also be beneficial to him." Thus, after Jack graduated from high school, he enrolled in college studies. His ambition was to become "a mechanical engineer."

The Second Neuropsychological Evaluation

Things, however, did not go well. Two years later, Jack was referred for a second neuropsychological evaluation (by a different psychologist). His grades at college deteriorated significantly, and he exhibited problems of "forgetfulness, distractibility, impulsivity, and poor judgment." He continued to live at home with his father and mother (an older brother was away at college). The psychologist's report noted that Jack "did poorly" in his classes, "failed to turn in most of his assignments," and "dropped several classes, and had to retake more than one class." The report further noted that "Jack had difficulty maintaining steady employment," "did not follow the rules at home," and has been "involved in multiple relationships with the opposite sex." This was totally "out of character" for him, compared to his "shyness" before the injury. The psychologist also reported "irresponsible behaviors," "conflicts with his parents," and "erratic" and "irritable" behaviors. The parents also complained about Jack's experiencing "sleep problems." This time, Jack himself complained of having "continuous headaches" and of being easily distracted. When confronted by the psychologist, Jack admitted that he engaged in "self-defeating behaviors" (by which he referred to his irresponsible behaviors, such as lying and engaging in illegal activities). Jack also admitted to having "mood swings" and to having a "negative view of the future." At the time of this evaluation, Jack was followed by a psychiatrist who prescribed two medications for him. Extensive psychometric tests and neurobehavioral observations yielded the following:

- *An estimated premorbid IQ within the high-average normal range (previously described as the "bright-normal range")*

- *Verbal processing speed, average to above average*

- *Intellectual functioning within the high-average range (verbal IQ = 112, 79 percentile; performance IQ = 117, 87 percentile)*

- *Better scores on visuomotor and visual pattern analytic tests and on mathematical tests*

- *Problems with tests that required "sustained concentration"*

- *In the executive functions area, performance that was "less efficient than during his earlier testing"*

- *That verbal fluency was found to be intact and no aphasic symptomatology was observed*

- *In the area of memory and learning, "overall memory functioning that was below what would be expected from him premorbidly"; that* "relatively low performance [levels] were observed in both verbal and visual memory tests"

■ In the emotional sphere and the assessment of his current personality, comments included in the report such as: "having difficulty self-monitoring and self-regulating his behavior," having concerns about his intellectual "dullness," being concerned about his "family discord," acknowledging feeling "depressed" and engaging (in what the psychologist labeled as) "hypomanic" and "amoral" behaviors.

■ That projective testing revealed "low self-esteem," "despair," "feeling that he has let others down," feeling "broken," "fearing that his ego resources [were] not adequate to meet the demands" of situations that he encountered, and having "limited frustration tolerance."

■ On the positive side, that Jack's assessment revealed "an adaptive capacity to cope, provided that the external stresses are not overwhelming" and that "despite his apparent lack of control and lack of accountability [Jack] felt guilty and remorseful for his (negative and self-destructive) actions"

■ That the psychologist felt that Jack's self-critical attitude may have also been provoked by feelings of loneliness and the fear that he lost his parents' love (hence—in the opinion of the psychologist—Jack's exaggerated "neediness" and his apparently frantic pursuit of relationships with females)

Among his many recommendations, the psychologist encouraged Jack (1) to seek intensive and ongoing physiatric and psychiatric support in an outpatient program, where "structure and environmental cuing are provided," and (2) to reduce his college course load and request tutorial help. At the insistence of his parents, Jack enrolled in an outpatient program near his home and was closely followed by a well- known physiatrist (who held regular consultations with the psychiatrist and the outpatient program's team members).

The Third Neuropsychological Evaluation

After Jack enrolled into the outpatient rehabilitation program, however, his adjustment problems became even more severe. He was then referred for yet a third neuropsychological evaluation. The third evaluation took place *about 3 years after Jack's motor vehicle accident. The following are the highlights of the extensive report:*

■ *During the clinical interview, Jack "began acting manicky" and declared that "[he] became [his] own authority," that he was not listening to anyone or "following rules of any kind." He acknowledged that his behavior could be symptomatic of an organic mood disorder, since previously he had been shy and not a particularly outgoing person.*

■ *Jack admitted that he had become increasingly "aggressive," "erratic," and "driven." He stated that he did not "feel depressed"; that he stayed out late (at times all night); that he "battled constantly" with his parents; and that when he became 18 years old, he "left home and stayed with friends." He admitted that at times he was "out of control." Yet, Jack also appeared to justify those behaviors as attempts "to be more independent."*

■ *Jack did not, however, try to justify his many impulsive, amoral, illegal, and defiant behaviors but had "explanations" for all of them.*

■ *During his interview, Jack admitted to having trouble "getting [himself] motivated for classes and school work" (he was still attending classes at college at the time). Nor was he motivated for many other activities. His leisure pursuits included "extreme sports" (hockey, skiing, snow boarding, fast driving). He claimed that he liked the "adrenalin rush" such activities caused, but that he also wished at times "to find [his] limits" because he tended "to overdo it."*

■ *Jack accepted that he had a "brain injury." He also acknowledged that he was having "a problem [living up to] people's expectations" of him. He felt that his problems were primarily motivational, or the result of "poor judgment and sometimes poor memory."*

■ *Jack expressed his dislike for the outpatient program and felt embarrassed being seen "in the company" of other brain-injured patients, feeling he had been in the program "far too long." He felt, however, that the medications that were prescribed for him "helped" him.*

■ *Jack admitted that he "used to" smoke marijuana and to drink alcohol, but claimed that he has been "clean for 1 ½ years."*

- He said that he preferred his father to become his "legal guardian" instead of an aunt who was appointed legal guardian during the preceding year.

- Jack cooperated during the testing and did not exhibit any "grossly inappropriate" behaviors.

Key Test Findings. *Jack was found to be "free from significant problems with concentration" while performing "structured tests," his verbal IQ was 106 (average) but his performance IQ was 125 (superior), his memory functions were average; his reasoning processes were "intact" (but weaker on verbal tests), and his executive functions were "excellent." The psychologist emphasized that while on formal tests, Jack's reasoning processes were good, in "unstructured [daily life] situations he was not exercising good judgment and sufficient self-control." Jack's personality assessment (by projective tests) indicated "an absence of psychosis or major thought disorder." While professing to have "few psychological problems" and "feeling generally happy," Jack's responses suggested that he had "difficulties establishing and maintaining satisfactory relationships." But, despite his overt problem behaviors, the psychologist also noted that Jack had some positive "inner resources" (such as emotional resiliency, the absence of a tendency to brood, and basic self-esteem).*

The third neuropsychological assessment confirmed most of the findings of the second psychologist. But the psychologist felt that although Jack's "façade of bravado and risk-taking behavior" were the obvious problems, his "amiability and yearning for approval and acceptance by others" were promising signs that were well worth "exploiting therapeutically." If only Jack could be helped to "better control his chaotic behavior and establish a greater rapport with his therapist," the psychologist felt that Jack could benefit from rehabilitative interventions.

Jack Applies for Entry into Our Program

Having reached the point of despair, Jack's parents consulted another doctor who recommended that they try to enroll their son into our program. The parents asked the opinion of the physiatrist who had been coordinating Jack's outpatient program. The physiatrist (who is familiar with our program) frankly told the parents that Jack was not yet "ready." But he nevertheless wished them "good luck" in their attempt to enroll Jack into our program. Thus, Jack and his mother came to New York to observe our program for 2 days and to be interviewed by one of the coauthors (YBY).

The Interview and the Initial Assessment of Jack

During the interview of Jack (in his mother's presence), he was "charming" and very complimentary about our program (which he observed as a visitor for 2 full days). He asserted that if he was accepted he would "do well" in our therapeutic community setting. (Jack was impressed by the attractiveness and the intellectual level of most of our patients and said that he felt "at home" in the company of such peers.) Jack's mother also expressed her hope that Jack would be accepted. She stated that if Jack would be enrolled in our program, she would close her legal practice, come to live with her son in New York, and attend regularly as Jack's "significant other." (About one-third to one-half of the significant others of any given patient group attend all of our daily program activities.) Since one of the out-of-town patients on our waiting list informed us that he could not come to New York (with his mother) until 6 months later, we accepted Jack in his place on two conditions: (1) that Jack undergo several days of testing and clinical observations, and (2) that he had to "fit in" in our therapeutic community and follow the "rules of conduct" in our program.

Results of Jack's Initial Evaluation

Cognitive and Neurobehavioral Findings. *On the first day of his initial assessment, Jack was clean-shaven, arrived appropriately dressed, and had gotten a haircut. He complied with all the examiners' requests and cooperated fully while being tested. He also behaved toward the other patients (most of whom later became his peers) in a friendly manner. On a comprehensive battery of tests, Jack was found to be*

- *Mildly impaired on tests of attention and concentration*

- *Mildly impaired on a test of visual analysis (Raven Progressive Matrixes)*

- *Severely impaired on a measure of higher-level convergent reasoning; moderately impaired on selected verbal tests of divergent reasoning*

- *In the 90th percentile (i.e., at the bottom of the superior-normal range) on a test of critical-evaluative thinking (which in his case was normal).*

- Impaired, however, on two verbal tests of executive functions, while on nonverbal tests of executive functions, within the normal range

Small-Group Interaction with a Peer Group. *In a formal, guided interview, in the presence of his peers and their significant others, Jack was friendly and came through as a likable person who was eager to join our program. He received excellent feedback from all the participants (all new candidates receive feedback after their interview). Thus, in spite of some doubts, we accepted Jack into our program. He commenced his intensive treatments 8 weeks later.*

The First Signs of Trouble and Our Response

Within days after commencing his training in our program, we received complaints from Jack's mother that

- *Jack insisted on staying out late at night (and lied to her about where he was).*

- *He was staying up until after midnight and communicating with "friends" on his cell phone (greatly exceeding the number of minutes that he was allowed for that purpose).*

- *His mother found in Jack's room an envelope with $3,000 (which, we strongly suspected, were the proceeds from selling drugs).*

At the program, however, Jack was compliant, except that he was observed taking cell phone calls during "bathroom breaks" or lunch hours.

Intervention

Our team worked out a plan of intervention. Jack and his mother were called in, and in the presence of the entire staff, Jack was presented with some "painful choices" by the program director (YBY). The presentation was conducted in a friendly atmosphere and in an empathic (i.e., "therapeutic") manner. The following is a (thematic, not verbatim) summary of the "plan."

Jack was reminded that his participation within our program was "satisfactory," that our team was "convinced" that he "possessed the potential for becoming, in time, rehabilitated." However, based on reports from his mother, our team was very much concerned about his ability to benefit from our program because of some of his recent behaviors.

Therefore, Jack had to choose between two painful alternatives: Either he returned to his home state immediately, or elected to stay and continue his treatments in our program. But, to continue, he had to abide by some conditions. The director (using paradoxical intention techniques) admitted that "most young people would find our conditions to be unacceptable" and, therefore, it would not be surprising if Jack "decided to leave our program immediately." The director then spelled out the conditions as follows: (1) Jack would have to return each day (after the program sessions) to the apartment that he and his mother shared; (2) stay in every night; (3) submit to a strict budget (including the number of phone calls he would be allowed to make); (4) socialize only with peers from our program, and if he desired to leave the apartment, he had to agree to being accompanied and supervised by his mother. Jack was also told that (5) staying up late at night was "out of the question," and if he had difficulties falling asleep, we would refer him to our consulting psychopharmacologist. Once again, Jack was told that "quite possibly" he may be unable to follow our demands "to the letter," and that "some people would describe them as a demand that he volunteer to live in a prison, with [his] mother acting as [his] jailer and our spy." Jack was also told that in case he decided to withdraw from our program, we would be "ready to accept [him] back" at a future time. But only if he would be willing to abide by our "draconian" rules. It was emphasized that we did not wish to inflict on him and his mother more suffering than they already had to endure, but we wished to test whether he had "what it takes" to "pay the price for your rehabilitation." To our surprise, Jack accepted our terms, stating that he "never quit any challenge in [his] life." He was then warmly congratulated for his "courage" and maturity."

Case Study 6 ("Liz")

Liz was 38 years old when she was referred to our program by a renowned neuropsychologist (who authored several highly thought-of books on brain injury). Liz was brought by her parents from South Africa to be evaluated by the referring psychologist. She is a multilingual (English, French, Afrikaner) white, attractive single woman. Her parents and three brothers are all high achievers and very successful in their respective careers. Liz herself completed 3 years of college but never worked.

Liz's medical history and personal life were very problematic: At the age of 3, she fell and injured her head, "became blue," needed mouth-to-mouth resuscitation, and suffered a parietal-occipital skull fracture. At the age of 10, she had meningitis with high fever and headaches. In addition, a history of depression was first diagnosed at age 15, and at the age of 16 there was an episode of self-mutilation with a knife. At the age of 20, there was a suicidal attempt with pill overdose. Liz also had a history of substance abuse (alcohol, ecstasy, cocaine).

At the age of 28, Liz sustained her second traumatic head injury, when, in a drunken state, she drove her car into a tree. She was unconscious for 3 days and incontinent. Upon regaining consciousness, Liz was confused and incoherent and was unable to walk because of her impaired balance. She suffered from double vision in her right eye, became easily fatigued, and had multiple cognitive deficits (including memory problems).

During the 10 years since her motor vehicle accident, Liz attempted to take various courses but never finished any of them. She attempted various jobs (as a waitress or a model) but was unable to embark on a successful vocational career. She was introduced to crack cocaine and prostituted herself for drugs. Her addiction-related behaviors caused her to be arrested and jailed twice; she has had five known seizures (presumed to be drug induced) and had several psychiatric hospitalizations.

When seen by the referring neuropsychologist, Liz claimed that she had been "free of any drugs and sober" for at least 8 months. (Her mother supported her in her claim. But, as we found out later, Liz's report concerning her sobriety was not totally accurate.)

Liz lived with her parents in Johannesburg. She was demoralized and very concerned about her inability to achieve a satisfactory career and to establish a "meaningful" personal life. At the time, she had a boyfriend in South Africa (a divorced Irish man). Liz's parents described the man to be a "nice enough" gentleman who seemed to genuinely care for Liz. But the parents were concerned about the fact that the man's close social friends spent much of their time drinking in bars, which (for obvious reasons) worried Liz's parents.

At our program, Liz underwent a comprehensive evaluation. The results revealed the following:

Liz's current IQ of 86 fell within the low-average range, which, on the basis of her mother's report that, before her first head injury, Liz was evaluated to have been an "extremely bright child," suggested significant decreases had taken place in her current intellectual efficiency.

Memory test results also suggested that Liz's current memory functions were "virtually certain" to be significantly below premorbid levels.

The test findings also suggested

- *Mild but clinically significant language deficits*

- *Mild but clinically significant impairments of her visual analytic abilities*

- *Moderate impairment of her new (verbal) learning ability*

- *Clinically significant attentional deficits (which, however, fluctuated between significant impairment, due to impulsivity, on one day and superior-normal levels of performance on the next)*

- *Severe executive functions deficits, consisting of impaired planning and organizing difficulties, impaired problem-solving abilities, and an inability to flexibly shift her thinking when called upon to consider some issues from different points of view*

The referring neuropsychologist found Liz to have "significant and widespread cognitive" deficits that were consistent with "bilateral diffuse central dysfunction with a particular impact on [her] frontolimbic structures and her right hemisphere." Our own findings suggested that our program may prove to be the "right place" for Liz. Thus, Liz applied for entry into our program and was accepted.

Outcome

Although Liz proved to be a challenging trainee, we have been most encouraged by her positive response to the treatments. After three cycles, she and her parents returned to South Africa. As of this writing, the reports from Liz and her parents were that she was making a satisfactory adjustment.

DVD Illustrations

Chapter 5 DVD, Volume 1

Sample 1: "Brendan", Group Interview

Sample 2: "Brendan", 1st Cycle Speech

Sample 3: Brendan, 5th Cycle Speech

Chapter 5 DVD, Volume 2

Sample 1: "Martha"

Sample 2: "Raquel"

Sample 3: "Jack"

Sample 4: "Liz"

Chapter 6 | *Starting a Treatment Cycle*

This chapter articulates the main clinical objective of the first few days at the start of a new treatment cycle. To illustrate how the various program activities (during the first 4 to 5 days) are designed to complement each other, excerpts of four of these videotaped program activities are presented in this chapter's companion DVD.

Overall Objectives of a New Cycle

Reduced to basics and simply stated, the overall objective during the first few days of a new cycle is to convey to the new trainees and their significant others (1) that they have become part of a special therapeutic community, (2) that their peer group is made up of individuals *who differ* in terms of their age, education, careers, and socioeconomic circumstances, (3) that they have just become part of an *exceptional program and part of a peer group of "privileged" people*, (4) that the staff of this program consists of highly *competent and trustworthy* professionals, and finally (5) that receiving intensive rehabilitative treatments in this program can also provide experiences of *drama and (occasionally) even fun (all of which takes place while they are learning about themselves and what they could or could not do).*

In the following sections, each of the foregoing points is further elucidated.

Membership in a "Therapeutic Community"

The sense that the trainee has just become part of a "therapeutic community" is conveyed by the highly structured and organized daily schedule, by the treatment "curriculum," by the fact that with few exceptions (e.g., personal counseling or some cognitive training "exercises") most of the program activities take place in small groups or "communal" settings, by the fact that (usually) about half of the members of the peer group are people who have already been in the program before (for one, or more, preceding treatment cycle), and by the special "rules of the house" (for example, "We do not give each other material gifts when we celebrate birthdays, but only verbal gifts.").

A Peer Group of Different People

The heterogeneity of the trainee peer group helps to bring out the best in each individual. The older, more accomplished (educationally, vocationally, and socioeconomically) trainees are challenged to act in their most "dignified" manner and to be role models to their younger peers in the way they deal with painful issues that all must face. These older trainees, in turn, are inspired by the way their younger peers struggle to achieve acceptance of their present reality, even though before their injury they have been unable to realize their personal and vocational "dreams." Both the older and younger *new* trainees have the opportunity to watch their "veteran" peers' commitment to the program and their implicit trust in the staff.

Feelings of "Exceptionableness"

The program staff deliberately (but subtly) encourages the trainees' belief that they belong to "the best program (of its kind) in the world"; that they were selected by the staff because (in the judgment of the staff) they possess the potential to overcome their dysfunctionality; and although they may not as yet fully understand the rationale for some of the treatments, they and their peers have enrolled into the program voluntarily, for their own sake, not just to please, or reassure, their families. Moreover, the staff also expects that until the trainees become fully educated about the staff's rationale for the different "exercises," they will follow professional advice on *trust*. Also, helping *to foster* feelings of *exceptionableness* is the fact that the program is open to visitation by rehabilitation professionals from all over the world, implying that the program is the focus of interest among professionals in the field.

The Staff as a Highly Competent Brain Trust

One of the aims is to create the impression, in the minds of the trainees and their significant others, that the program staff consists of highly competent and experienced professionals. By working together as a team they function as a Brain Trust. To help create this impression, the staff adopts a plain-speaking style. (For example, "We call a brain injury what it is—a tragedy!" Or, "We will always tell you the truth, but with compassion.") The impression that the program staff consists of competent, hard-working, and reliable professionals is further reinforced by the staff's "modesty." Several examples will suffice: "Although every one of us is well trained and informed, alone we can still, at times, make mistakes. But by consulting with each other we pool our experiences and knowledge, reducing the chances that we will make big mistakes." Or, "when we don't know something, you can trust that we will always ask the advice of colleagues who are more knowledgeable than we are."

Drama and Fun

To ease the tension that is, unavoidably, created by the fast-moving and intellectually challenging program activities, the staff resorts to the liberal use of humor and to the creation of a sense of drama and (pleasing) surprise. Several examples illustrate this: In a group "exercise," the designated leader addressed a young trainee: "Now we would like to hear from Ms. Philippine Islands." Or while soliciting a comment from an older trainee—an anthropology professor—the leader said: "And what does the professor think?" At another time, during the last session in a week (e.g., on a Thursday), the designated leader closed the session with these words: "Now go home in peace, recharge your batteries, and come back on Monday, back to the salt mines, so that we may torture you some more…" Thus, by judiciously balancing hard and intensive work with surprise, drama, and humor, tension is kept within tolerable (i.e., manageable) limits.

A Crescendo of Program Activities Aimed at "Setting the Right Tone"

The first four days into a new cycle of treatment are devoted to creating the "right impressions" about the program as well as the staff. Activities are planned by the staff in such a way as to cumulatively bring about the desired impressions. Four such activities (spread out over 4 to 5 consecutive days) are briefly described below and illustrated by (selected) excerpts from actual videotaped sessions in the companion DVD of this chapter.

Self-Introductions

On the first day, once all trainees, their significant others, members of the staff, and visitors (if any are present on that day) are seated, all are asked by the designated leader of that session to introduce themselves. The leader is first to demonstrate how this is done. When members of the staff introduce themselves, they make a special effort not to assume a "professional" demeanor and to come through as "interesting and regular" people. The leader asks the trainees as well: "Do not tell us, at this point, how you were injured. There will be enough opportunities for that. Just tell us what you would like the people here to know about you in this first meeting." Significant others, and visitors, are also asked to briefly introduce themselves. This first, self-introductory session is usually accompanied by much laughter and serves to heighten the interest of the new and old members of the "therapeutic community" about things to come.

The "Philosophy" of the Program Articulated

In a session that follows (also on the first day), another member of the staff is designated to lead a discussion about the "philosophy of the program." The "philosophy" of the program is defined as: "how the staff views the purposes of the rehabilitation process and the staff's attitude toward the trainees." "Veteran" trainees, including selected previous trainees of the program (who are also invited to attend this session), are encouraged to articulate, in their own words, based on their own personal experiences, what the staff mean, for example, when they make assertions such as: "In this program, you don't have to leave your dignity outside when you enter." Or, "Here we believe that the consumers (i.e., the trainees) deserve to be told the truth—with compassion, of course—because in our opinion, telling them the truth is the truest way of showing respect for our trainees." Significant others of "veteran" trainees are also encouraged to take an active part in the discussion about the "philosophy" of the program. Similarly, the other members of the staff raise their hand, to be recognized by the designated leader, and express their own points of view. This contributes to the impression that people in this "community" are "partners" who deliberate together, but in an orderly and disciplined manner, so that everyone's opinion will be heard.

"Peer Counselors" Build an Atmosphere of Hope

To provide the trainees with actual "role models" who achieved success in their rehabilitation, and thus create an atmosphere of hope, "peer counselors" (ex-trainees) are "debriefed' in the presence of the trainees and their significant others (such "debriefing" takes place on the third or fourth day). Trainees are free to ask the "peer counselors" questions about their experiences, feelings, and current lives.

The Two-Minute "Exercise"

Usually on the second day, the designated leader explains the rationale for a particular "exercise" which is to follow:

> Each of you trainees will be called upon to take the "hot seat" and, upon getting a cue from the designated "timekeeper," deliver a two-minute self-introduction. To do that, each one of you will have to plan what to say and how to say it, within two minutes. In life, we are all faced with situations in which we must respond, "on the spot," or say what we want to say, briefly and in an understandable manner. This is not easy to do and in this program we will practice how to do it effectively.

The leader then adds (reassuringly): "For some people, 2 minutes is not enough time to say what they have in mind. For others, on the other hand, 2 minutes is too much time. Either way, there is no pass or fail grade. Just do the best you can and when the time is up, go back to your seat." Both the trainees and their significant others find this exercise to be dramatic and quite interesting. For the staff, the 2-minute self-introduction by each trainee provides additional diagnostic information concerning the adequacy of the trainee's "executive" skills (in the context of interpersonal communications, when time is limited and a successful communicator must find a way to state the essentials). This "exercise," at the very beginning of the treatment cycle, also conveys the "message" that this program will be devoted to "serious" work, under the leadership of a well- coordinated "coaching staff."

DVD Illustrations

Chapter 6 DVD

Volume 1 presents video clips illustrating the initial self-introductions of the members of the "therapeutic community".

Volume 2 presents edited video clips illustrating the introduction of the philosophy of the program.

Volume 3 presents edited video clips of the introduction of peer counselors to the therapeutic community.

Volume 4 presents the first "hot seat" experience.

Chapter 7 | *Exploiting the "Halo" Effects from Professional Visits*

This chapter outlines the principal "halo" effects of visits by professionals who have observed our program, and it illustrates (see excerpts on the chapter's DVD) interactions of several renowned professionals in the field of neuropsychological rehabilitation with our "therapeutic community."

In earlier chapters we pointed out that in the "therapeutic community" the *composition of the trainee peer group*, the *complementary nature* of the various *programmatic elements*, and the explicitly as well as implicitly expressed *staff attitude* all exert strong influences on the individual trainee in our program as well as on his or her significant others.

Because of the reputation of our program as being a model of the (Goldsteinian) holistic approach to neuropsychological rehabilitation, the program is frequently visited by medical and paramedical professionals from all over the world. Among these visitors are some of the most prominent psychologists in our field.

The open-visitation policy is yet another component of the aggregate of clinical influences, which shape both the attitude (as well as the behaviors) of the trainees. Several of the "halo" effects of visits by prominent professionals in the field are deliberately exploited by the staff. These are outlined in the following sections.

"Halo" Effects of Visits by Prominent Professionals

The visits are incorporated into the daily schedule. Whenever such visits are planned, the staff programs special sessions that make possible the direct interactions between the visiting professional and the members of the "therapeutic community." Typically, such sessions are chaired by a senior staff member and involve:

- The introduction of the visitor

- A request that the visiting professional share with the "community" his or her impressions, observations, or thoughts about the program

- A request, by the leader, that each trainee articulate, for the benefit of the visitor, a question concerning the nature of the program, or his or her thoughts or feelings about the program, or his or her progress in rehabilitation up to that point; trainees are asked to "think about the question," prepare written "talking points," and when "your turn comes," to articulate their thoughts concisely and "as clearly as you can"

- Solicitation of comments from the significant others and the staff as well

- A request that each trainee ask the visitor an *appropriate question*.

- Direct interactions between the visitor and certain individuals

Experience has shown that such exchanges enhance the "esprit de corps" of the trainees and their feeling that they belong to an "elite" group of rehabilitants. These exchanges also contribute to their sense of self-esteem, when they realize that the distinguished visitors are impressed by their high morale, thoughtfulness, and articulateness.

DVD Illustrations

Four illustrations are provided in Chapter 7 DVD.

Volume 1: Professor Barbara Wilson's (England) Visit

Prior to the author's (YBY) arrival with Professor Wilson, the trainees discussed the benefits they derive from visits by distinguished professionals. Volume 1 presents the opinions of two trainees. Then, following the introduction of Professor Wilson to the group, three trainees describe the specific problem that each had been working on overcoming at the time.

Volume 2: Professor Anne-Lise Christensen's (Denmark) and Professor Nicole Von Steinbuchel's (Germany) Visit

The two visitors are introduced. Then, several trainees describe the specific problem area (described by their personal poster) that was, at the time, the target of intensive remedial interventions.

Volume 3: Professor George Prigatano's (US–Arizona) Visit

After Professor Prigatano is introduced, ten trainees provide their self-definition (also known as a description of their reconstituted "ego identity" following rehabilitation).

Volume 4: Professor Dan Hoofien's (Israel) Visit

Professor Hoofien shares with the community his impressions after observing the program for a full week.

Chapter 8   *Fostering Awareness and Self-Understanding*

This chapter restates the importance of awareness and self-understanding in the neuropsychological rehabilitative process, describes five specific remedial or therapeutic activities that were designed to promote self-understanding, and illustrates these techniques in videotaped excerpts on the DVD for this chapter.

Significance of Self-Understanding

Briefly restated, the central clinical objectives of holistic neuropsychological rehabilitation are to help the brain-injured individual to compensate for his or her neurobehavioral deficits and to optimize his or her cognitive and interpersonal functioning. This includes applying compensatory skills and strategies, acquired in the setting of the rehabilitative program, in his or her functional life. In other words, integrating these compensatory skills with his or her other functional repertoires. The ultimate aim is to help the individual trainee find meaning in life after rehabilitation.

Kurt Goldstein has taught us that this clinical objective cannot be achieved without the brain-injured individual's voluntary and equanimous acceptance of the fact that certain aspects of lifestyle, or career objectives, that he or she pursued before the brain injury may now become impossible to attain. Therefore, the individual will now have to give up (voluntarily and with equanimity) pursuing unattainable goals and concentrate on achieving those functional goals that still remain possible to attain under the circumstances.

The requirement of voluntary (and equanimous) acceptance of what will or will not be possible to achieve, due to the limitations that have been imposed by the brain injury, necessitates the thorough education of the person about the nature and consequences of the various deficits that he or she sustained as a result of the brain injury. This means developing a full awareness and understanding of one's present and future needs (in terms of assistance or guidance) and of one's capabilities, as well the need to accept one's limitations. For only awareness and self-understanding can and will motivate the individual to engage—wholeheartedly—in the sustained process of rehabilitative interventions, under the guidance of trained professionals.

Techniques That Promote Self-Understanding

We have already pointed out that each program element was designed and coordinated with the others in mind, so that the effects of each would complement and reinforce the effects of the others. As experience has shown, these coordinated activities can cumulatively produce the desired outcomes. The promotion of awareness and self-understanding, therefore, makes it necessary to deal *during any* specific remedial or therapeutic activity in which an individual trainee is engaged with issues such as: (1) *motivating* the trainee to actively and fully engage in the task at hand (by pointing out to the trainee the relevance of the particular activity to the enhancement of the trainee's functional competence), (2) ensuring that the trainee's *attention and concentration functions* are optimally focused throughout the training "exercise" (thus making possible the learning, retention, and the transfer of learned compensations from the program into functional life contexts), (3) ensuring that the remedial routine is *broken down into subroutines* and the trainee is provided with adequate performance-facilitating cues (to ensure the mastery and habituation of compensatory skills), (4) *adequately managing* the trainee's *emotional frustration* or cognitive difficulties (that interfere with the orderly learning process), and (5) and consistently *interpreting* for the trainee the *meaning and functional implications* of his or her progress. Interventions aimed at fostering awareness and self-understanding thus take place in all the structured program activities as shown in Table 8.1.

Table 8.1. Emphasis on Self-Understanding during the Various Formal (Structured) Program Sessions

Program session	Description
▨ Orientation	Trainees rehearse daily their individualized "posters."
▨ Interpersonal group exercise	Among the other concerns, all group exercises involve the systematic focusing by the staff on the trainee's self-understanding.
▨ Cognitive remedial training	Self-understanding is integrated with the didactic aspects of the cognitive training.
▨ "Community" hour	All "community" sessions emphasize self-understanding as well.
▨ Personal counseling	Verification of the trainee's self-understanding is likewise a primary focus during personal counseling sessions.
▨ Oral "report card"	Verification of the trainee's comprehension and self-understanding is a key requirement during these exercises.

DVD Illustrations

Chapter 8 DVD

Volume 1 presents edited video clips illustrating how, in a group exercise, a trainee defines a personality quality that will prevent her from becoming, in the future, a bitter, self-defeated person.

Volume 2 presents edited video clips illustrating how three trainees describe their particular difficulty with memory as they experience it during their daily lives.

Volume 3 presents edited video clips illustrating how several trainees and significant others assess why the program has been helpful in their case.

Volume 4 presents edited video clips illustrating a trainee's description of (his) gains from the treatments. (Taking stock)

Volume 5 presents edited video clips from a special role-playing "exercise" (in which the trainee interviews herself, as role-played by a staff member).

Chapter 9

Facilitating Compensation in the Cognitive Domains of Functioning

This chapter (1) reiterates the essentials of cognitive remedial intervention in the context of the "therapeutic community" program, (2) describes five specific remedial techniques designed to ameliorate deficiencies in various aspects of cognitive functioning, and (3) illustrates these techniques via excerpts of videotaped "exercises."

Essentials of Cognitive Remedial Intervention

As already outlined in earlier chapters, remedial and therapeutic interventions in the cognitive sphere take place in a series of overlapping and coordinated stages. These stages commence with interventions aimed at (1) *engaging* (i.e., motivating) the trainees to participate in the rehabilitative endeavor; (2) *ameliorating disinhibitive* or *adynamic* phenomena (to make possible for learning to take place); (3) addressing deficits in perceptual-cognitive and information-processing functions (thus enhancing memory and retention of learning); (4) *enhancing* convergent, divergent, and "executive" functioning—*higher level reasoning abilities*—which lead to acceptance of one's limitations and to the reconstitution of one's ego-identity and ultimately result in (5) the *optimal postrehabilitation adjustment* of the person.

Five Types of Cognitive Remedial Training

In the following sections, we describe five specific types of cognitive remedial training procedures, ranging from remedial procedures designed to ameliorate basic attentional deficits, all the way to procedures designed to improve higher level reasoning functions.

Improving Basic Attentional Functions

K., a 72-year-old investment banker from Cairo, Egypt (with a PhD from MIT, an MBA from Harvard University, and an engineering degree from Cambridge University), fell down a flight of stairs and sustained a number of severe cognitive deficits. Two of K.'s most prominent deficits were a frontal lobe unawareness syndrome and severe adynamia (problems in initiating words or actions).

Simultaneously with vigorous interventions designed to make K. *aware* of the consequences of his injury and to help him *initiate* more (and therefore be less dependent on his wife and adult daughters), he underwent systematic training to improve his attention and concentration functions.

C., a 37-year-old Wall Street analyst (with an MBA degree) suffered a cardiac arrest, which resulted in multiple cognitive, neurobehavioral, and emotional problems. Among his many deficits in basic and higher level reasoning functions, C.'s expressive aphasia posed a major problem. His moderately severe cognitive deficits were exacerbated by C.'s agitated depression over his wife's declared intention to divorce him, coupled with the emotional "blow" of being let go by his employer.

K. and C. were matched up as training partners on a computerized hierarchy of remedial training designed to improve their concentration.

Training to Improve Integration of Perceptual-Cognitive and Constructional Abilities

Having successfully completed her remedial training to improve attention and concentration, as well as training on various visual information–processing tasks, R. (see "Raquel" in Chapter 5 underwent advanced intensive training in the planning and the construction of block designs. The training module consisted of designs of increasing complexity.

Training to Improve Convergent and Divergent Reasoning Ability

Following the initial stages of her remedial interventions (aimed at improving awareness and self-understanding of attentional functions), J., a 63-year-old professor of anthropology and published novelist (who underwent radical treatments for a brain tumor), received systematic training designed to improve her convergent and divergent reasoning abilities.

"Exercises" Designed to "Spark" Imagination

L., a 24-year-old Japanese college student (who prior to his injury was enrolled at an American Ivy League university) was matched up with R. Both underwent special "exercises" designed to "spark" their imagination. The purpose of these exercises was to induce both L. and R. to "project" alternative imaginary "scenarios" for pictorial stimuli (i.e., producing alternative "stories" and expressing these stories by using consensually validated vocabularies). These exercises were conducted by an advanced trainee, "Laura," who prior to her traumatic brain injury was employed as a creative director at a world-renowned publisher.

Role-Playing a "Junior Psychologist"

In an afternoon cognitive session, devoted to enhancing her interpersonal communication skills, J. engaged in a guided dialogue with "Laura." The topic of the dialogue was: "How do you overcome neurofatigue?" (See this chapter's DVD, Volume 5.)

DVD Illustrations

Chapter 9 DVD

Volume 1 presents edited video clips illustrating remedial training in the domain of attention-concentration.

Volume 2 presents edited video clips illustrating remedial training to improve construction of block designs.

Volume 3 presents edited video clips illustrating remedial training to improve convergent reasoning ability.

Volume 4 presents edited video clips illustrating remedial training in "sparking" to improve the imagination.

Volume 5 presents edited video clips illustrating a dialogue with a peer.

Chapter 10   *Contributions of Significant Others*

This chapter reiterates the important roles played by significant others, as "partners" and active participants in the complementary activities of the therapeutic community; describes three of those roles and illustrates them with videotaped excerpts.

Roles of Significant Others in the Therapeutic Community

As pointed out earlier, the ubiquitous presence (by a third to a half of significant others [SOs]) in *all the program* activities provides excellent role models of wise, empathic, and respectful adults to the trainees. Also, because of their deep and long-standing emotional ties with their own family member (who is a trainee in the program) and by acting, vicariously, as SOs to nonfamily program trainees, the significant others reinforce the trust of community members in the staff's professional competence, honesty, and dedication. Hence, the significant others contribute to trainees' acceptance of the staff's leadership and inspire them to work hard toward achieving the necessary equanimous acceptance of their predicament.

But, significant others also benefit from their active participation in the program: The open acknowledgment of the significant others that they, too, *must learn, by observing the staff,* how to interact with their loved one in such a way that will *bring out the best* in the trainee (i.e., that the trainee will not feel either "infantilized" or "bossed" by the significant other) will help the significant others to become effective home "coaches" and advisors. In this way, the significant other enhances the trainee's rehabilitation—by fostering the trainees' willingness to learn from the staff and to follow their advice. The significant others, thus, become "allies" of the staff as well as willing "students." Another important result of the involvement of significant others in the program is that they, too, can learn to understand how the brain injury has impacted the life of their loved one; what can or cannot be achieved by rehabilitation; and how they can best assist their (chronologically adult) loved one, without "infantilizing" or "insulting" or provoking his or her resentment.

DVD Illustrations Chapter 10 DVD

Volume 1 presents the feedback of several S.O.'s to J.

Background

At the end of his fourth treatment cycle, J. (see Chapter 5, "Jack") received his "oral report card" in front of the entire "community." During this cycle, J. shared an apartment with his brother. This arrangement was by mutual agreement among all concerned. The intention was to provide J. with a "transitional" phase in his rehabilitation. From the omnipresent supervision and home "coaching" of his mother, J. transitioned to the less rigorous (but still omnipresent) advice (and supervision) of his brother. The understanding was that, if all went well during this cycle, J. could look forward to living on his own while he attended the fifth and sixth cycles in our program. (J.'s goal was to become totally independent in his living arrangements.)

After receiving his "oral report card," J. critiqued his own performance and received feedback from his peers, his brother, and the staff. Then, four "veteran" significant others, who followed J.'s progress from the time he initially enrolled into our program, provided him with their own feedback.

Volume 2 presents edited video clips of end-of-cycle going away wishes by S.O.'s

Background

During a final (end-of-cycle) community session, three outgoing "post-doctoral" fellows (who completed their training in our program) and two program trainees (who "graduated" and were about to return to their respective homes) received going away "best wishes" from all members of the community. As part of these "best wishes", the comments of several significant others are presented).

Volume 3 presents the end-of-cycle party "speech" of an S.O.

Background

At the conclusion of each end-of-cycle ("graduation") party, a significant other is asked to deliver a brief "speech" on his or her behalf and on behalf of all the significant others.

Chapter 11 *Managing Interferences with the Treatment Process*

In the previous chapters, we attempted to describe (and by means of companion DVDs to illustrate) how in a "therapeutic community" such as ours the structure, the curriculum, and the specific remedial and therapeutic interventions were interwoven in such a way that each aspect of the program complemented and reinforced the effects of the others.

Earlier, we attempted to show that the mutually complementary nature of the different program features made it possible to engage, to render malleable to treatments, and to ultimately rehabilitate even a number of initially hard-to-reach and problematic individuals. Our extensive clinical experiences have convinced us that in our "therapeutic community" setting, such problematic, brain-injured individuals proved able to respond well, even though they did not in more conventional neurorehabilitative programs.

However, to facilitate the sought-after transformations of attitudes, feelings, and behaviors of brain-injured people requires an appropriate mechanism for dealing effectively with the inevitable interferences with the "smooth" progress of the treatment of certain individuals, and with "crises" that often occur. In our program that mechanism is what came to be called by staff the "special poster session." The term "special poster session" originated from the fact that, during such clinical sessions, colorful posters are used in outlining key "talking points" or presenting explanatory diagrams.

Special "poster sessions" are tailor designed to fit the particular situation at hand. Such sessions take place by special invitation and are attended by the particular trainee in question, with or without the significant others, and the staff. On occasion, poster sessions are held only with significant others if and when the staff is concerned that the trainee may be traumatized or demoralized by participating in the poster session.

While preparing for a poster session, special attention is paid to questions such as

- How to introduce the problem at hand?

- How do the trainee or the significant others feel toward the staff, and how knowledgeable are they about the rationale for the various clinical interventions?

- What are the personalities of the trainee and the significant others, and what manner of presentation would most likely establish the "right" frame of mind and the desirable "atmospherics" for the serious deliberations that will have to follow?

Three specific examples of poster sessions are briefly described in the following sections. Each is illustrated by edited videotaped excerpts from the actual sessions.

Example 1: "Adele"

Adele's parents were invited to meet with the staff. The questions were whether or not Adele had reached her final "plateau" in our outpatient day program setting, and whether or not the parents should consider placing her in a long-term residential facility.

Background

Before her injury, Adele was a high school graduate, of average intelligence, who was employed full-time as a receptionist at a computer school. She was a "happy," socially active, "party-loving" young woman, who was well liked by her peers and who had an intimate relationship with a young musician boyfriend. Both Adele and her parents expected that she would eventually marry her boyfriend.

At the age of 21, Adele sustained severe brain injuries when a car, driven by a drunk driver, collided head on with Adele's car.

At the scene of the accident, Adele was found comatose with a rating of 3 on the Glasgow Coma Scale. She remained unconscious for the following 30 days.

Upon regaining consciousness, Adele was diagnosed as exhibiting symptoms of a severe frontal lobe syndrome including

- *Very impaired attention and concentration*

- *Dense hemiparesis*

- *A lack of concern and lack of embarrassment over her inappropriate behaviors*

- *Dramatic alterations in her preinjury personality*

- *"Issues of sexuality"*

Adele was described as having been unaware of the degree to which her premorbid cognitive and interpersonal functions became "degraded" by her significant frontal lobe damage. She attended several inpatient and outpatient rehabilitation programs for 2 years subsequent to her injury. But she remained a very problematic and functionally incapacitated young woman. By the age of 24, she returned home to her parents.

She was evaluated at our facility and was soon enrolled into our program, where, subsequently, she attended for four treatment cycles (about 2 years).

Initially, Adele was friendly, but very disinhibited. She constantly interrupted her examiners or "coaches" midsentence. (When this was called to her attention, she apologized for being "rude.") She was also unaware of the degree to which her injury rendered her dysfunctional, both in carrying out her daily activities and cognitively. She expressed "certainty" that she would "soon" be able to return to her preinjury work and marry her boyfriend (who continued to support her and frequently attended the program as a significant other). Her garrulous friendliness was accompanied by childlike questions, such as "Am I not your sweetest patient?" And she frequently demanded that she be hugged and told "how sweet" she was.

Although she complied and readily engaged in various cognitive remedial "exercises," Adele quickly "got bored" and became restless. But after "coaxing," she reengaged. Cognitively, her deficits ran the gamut from impulsively blurting out whatever came to her mind (but never expressing hostile or hurtful words), attentional, visual-perceptual, and memory problems, to higher level reasoning impairments (including deficits in her convergent reasoning, divergent reasoning, and executive functions).

However, when exhorted to "become serious and productive" and assisted by facilitatory cueing techniques, Adele often surprised the staff and her peers by her smart and insightful comments.

Gradually, she became more self-controlled during the program (raised her hand to be recognized and allowed to speak, provided appropriate feedback to her peers, willingly refrained from smoking during cognitive or group sessions, returned to classes after lunch breaks). At home, she increasingly complied with her parents by needing less coaxing or pressuring to take showers, to put on appropriate clothing, groom herself, and to generally behave toward visiting friends and family as a "polite young woman." Thus, Adele became a "civilized" 24-year-old woman, to the delight of her parents and her loyal boyfriend.

Unfortunately, two problems remained recurrent. First, from time to time (without apparent situational "provocations") Adele reverted back to some of her "old" maladaptive and recalcitrant behaviors (for example, refusing to shower, becoming "lazy," as her parents described it, or refusing to help her mother set the table).

In total, Adele underwent four treatment cycles in our program. During the first three cycles, she received intensive remedial interventions coupled with personal counseling and conjoint family counseling. During the fourth cycle, Adele was tested—both at our program facility as well as at an office at our medical center—to ascertain (1) whether or not she was capable of executing some aspects of lower level clerical tasks; (2) the extent to which she was able to work, without the constant physical presence of a work supervisor; and (3) the degree to which she was capable of being productive (i.e., how much work she was able to produce compared to an average paid employee who performed the same tasks). These work explorations revealed that Adele had the potential to become eventually vocationally engaged, albeit in a lower level clerical capacity. However, although when coached, supervised, and supported—at the program as well at home—Adele adjusted satisfactorily (for example, she became "disciplined", performed adequate daily self-care and hygiene tasks, and accepted "coaching" and reminders from her parents), the fact that she remained prone to lapses throughout her fourth cycle caused concern.

Second, Adele still had the persistent problem that she was unable to resist, or postpone, some strong impulses. For example, she ate the ice cream that belonged to a member of the staff. On another occasion, she carelessly crossed a highway, nearly getting hit by a car, when she "remembered" that she must buy a birthday card for her boyfriend.

Her persistent lapses, though only occasional, and her inability to resist strong urges prompted the question of whether or not Adele had attained the "final plateau" in our therapeutic community setting.

While, for obvious psychological reasons, her personal counselor did not spell out to Adele her future predicament (if her lapses kept recurring) in quite those stark terms, she was made aware of her situation in therapeutic terms. It is of interest, therefore, to see how, with the help of her counselor, Adele expressed her understanding in her speech at the end of the fourth-cycle party. Her speech follows.

End-of-Cycle Personal Statement

Although I'm completing my rehabilitation in this program, I know that rehabilitation is not over. The staff believes that I'm ready to test whether I can reliably apply my strategies to ALL aspects of my life, outside the program. I've worked extremely hard to overcome the effects of my severe frontal lobe injury and to become a competent woman.

I've learned that discontinuity, or gaps in awareness and memory, causes me to forget to use my compensations "in the moment." I'm also trying very hard to practice self-monitoring so I come on "just right"—not too strong or fast. Seeking feedback and coaching are my most critical strategies.

In this cycle, I've experienced many "ups and downs." I've learned that "talking the talk" is easy, but "walking the walk" is not. My motivation fluctuates from day to day (especially on Mondays). But I'm proud to say I've made slow and steady progress in overcoming many interferences in my life.

Sometimes, I feel sad and fearful; I wish my life was the way it used to be. Unfortunately, these thoughts cause me to "hide under the covers" and slow down my progress. My family and friends are worried I might not be able to get back "on track."

Recently, in my work trial, I've begun to feel hopeful. I love reading and singing songs to preschool children at the Rusk Institute. Their faces light up my day. Some have limited language or physical skills; nevertheless, they find a way to have fun. I love contributing to their day because they teach me how to embrace the joy of my life. Most of all, they teach me to have courage to do what's hardest.

I have my whole life ahead of me. I have to remember how good I feel when I apply the effort and do things the right way. Only when I habituate all of my strategies will I know how far I can go.

I thank my family, especially my Mom and Mike, for putting their lives on hold for me. I hope that you can begin focusing on your own future. Thank you, Tracey, for giving me so much of your time and patience. Thank you, Eric, for being my best friend and always being there for me. I love each and every one of you so much. Also, I'd like to thank the staff, my peers, and SOs for supporting me in my journey.

Thank you for listening.

Preparing for the Poster Session with Adele's Parents'

Who are the parents? *Gloria and Mike were highly intelligent individuals who*

- *Implicitly trusted the staff*

- *Were very grateful for what had already been accomplished with their daughter in four cycles*

- *Were attached to the other significant others, and at least one of them attended the program almost daily*

- *Followed through skillfully with all of the staff's suggestions for how to "coach" and manage Adele at home*

What should be the introductory remarks and the manner in which they should be delivered so that the parents would be best prepared to discuss with the staff the possibility of placing Adele in a residential facility?

It was decided that the introductory remarks should:

1. *Reiterate, in simple terms, the typical sequelae of frontal lobe injuries*

2. *Reiterate the underlying rationale of rehabilitative interventions in frontal lobe–injured individuals and how it is possible to determine whether or not the treatments proved effective in their daughter's case*

3. *Briefly explain the idea of plateaus in the acquisition of skills*

Chapter 11 DVD, Volume 1, presents edited excerpts of the introductory comments that preceded the deliberations.

Resolution

Adele's parents decided (sadly) to seek an appropriate residential facility for their daughter. The staff promised to help them persuade Adele—if necessary—that it would be in her best interest to accept enrolling at a residential facility.

Outcome

After a search and visits by the parents to several residential facilities, an appropriate one was located. Surprisingly, to the great relief of all concerned, Adele accepted, without arguments, to enter that program. A festive "going away" community session was dedicated to Adele. She received expressions of good wishes from our entire community. Then, from time to time Adele made phone calls informing us how well she was doing at the new facility. And, her parents, who became attached to the significant others and our staff, continued to attend the weekly sessions of the significant others and the midcycle and the end-of-cycle parties.

Example 2: "Brendan"

In Chapter 5, "Brendan" was described as the recalcitrant type of trainee. He completed five successful treatment cycles in our program. During the first two cycles, Brendan and his mother resided in a rented apartment near our program facility. During the third cycle, his mother returned to Texas, part of the time, to manage her various businesses, while one of her employees (a calm and fatherly gentleman whom Brendan liked and respected) took the mother's place as the "resident" significant other. During the fourth cycle, Brandon's brother (a recently graduated college student) came to stay with Brendan at the rented apartment (the mother came from Texas every few weeks, for short visits with both of her sons). During the fifth and six cycles, Brendan's mother returned to stay with him (full-time) until he was finally discharged from the program.

Throughout his stay in New York, Brendan had numerous "rebellions," during which he "threatened" to leave the program. But each time he was persuaded to stay and to continue his rehabilitation. Until the next "rebellion" occurred.

Among his other remarkable accomplishments as a program trainee, Brendan had learned to control his fierce temper outbursts. (He was regularly followed by our consulting psychopharmacologist and "optimally" medicated by him for his seizure disorder.) In addition, Brendan became a highly responsible, competent, and productive "worker" at the NYU print shop. He was well liked by his supervisors and derived great pleasure (and pride) from his very successful work trials.

One weekend, while visiting one of his male peers at the program (who also resided with his mother in the same building), Brandon beat up his peer because (as he later complained) he was "provoked" by "things that [his peer] said." We prevailed upon the peer's mother not to press charges against Brendan and promised to "deal with the problem" ourselves. Thus, with the help of his personal counselor, Brendan made restitution for his violent response to the mother of his peer, apologized to the entire "community," and wrote an effective letter to the peer whom he assaulted.

The staff had decided that a "poster session" should also be held. The concern was that Brendan's tendency to express anger, by physical violence, even though only on rare occasions, threatened his successful adjustment when he returned home to Texas.

Considerations in Preparing for the "Poster Session"

1. *How should the program director get across to Brendan his care and concern for him (Brendan loved and respected the director) and the fact that the staff was concerned about Brendan's proneness to express anger by physical violence (which the staff felt might endanger his ultimate rehabilitation)? At the same time, the aim was not to convey a sense of panic, or "gloom and doom."*

2. *What psychological "leverage" will be the most likely to engage Brendan's feelings as well as to mobilize his determination to overcome this vulnerability of his?*

Resolution

The poster session proved to be very successful. Brendan resumed his work trial and thereafter advised other peers (in crisis) to follow in his footsteps as a "believer" ("because these guys know what they are doing!")

Outcome

After his "graduation" from our program, Brendan returned to Texas; became the "manager" of one of his mother's businesses; took up living with an attractive girlfriend in an apartment of his own (with the intention of marrying her "soon"); and came to visit our program, at regular intervals, with his mother and "fiancé." He is received by the "community," on each of his visits, as a returning "hero."

Example 3: "Jack"

In Chapter 5 Jack was also described as one of the four problematic trainees who responded very positively to our "therapeutic community" setting. But his adjustment was not easy. It required dramatic interventions from time to time.

Jack completed five treatment cycles in our program. During the first two cycles, he was closely supervised by his mother (whom we humorously called his "jailer"); in the third cycle, which was termed his "transitional" cycle, Jack was guided and supervised by his brother; and during the fourth and fifth cycles, he lived alone while attending college classes and attempting to develop an acceptable ("normal") lifestyle as a socially active college student.

During his stay in New York, Jack was the recipient of three "poster sessions." The first poster session addressed the issue of Jack's progress toward reliably controlling unacceptable behaviors while away from the program. The second poster session was devoted to the identification of two main "obstructions" in Jack's path toward achieving his potential for rehabilitation. And the third poster session took place at the end of the third cycle. It addressed the question of whether or not Jack and his parents felt ready and able to take the risk of letting Jack live alone and to begin to realize (safely!) his yearning to be independent and his own "supervisor."

This chapter's DVD presents edited segments of.

> *These poster sessions were intended (a) to enhance Jack's trust in our staff and (b) to make his parents psychologically ready to consider (despite their many previous letdowns) the admittedly risky proposition of allowing Jack to live alone in New York while he still attended our program.*

Resolution

After lengthy deliberations, Jack's parents consented (with poorly disguised trepidations) to allow Jack to reside by himself in his apartment, manage his housekeeping chores; take care of his meals, adopt "healthy sleep habits," live within a reasonable budget as well as honestly account for his expenditures, and balance his college studies with acceptable recreational activities and a "healthy" social life. (By now, Jack had an attractive, intelligent and caring female college classmate as a girlfriend whom he, from time-to-time, invited to attend some of our program activities.)

Outcome

At the end of his fifth cycle, Jack returned to his Midwestern hometown where he continued his quest for independent living, pursued college studies, and received ongoing personal counseling from a local psychologist.

Periodically, Jack as paid a visit to our program with his girlfriend. His mother resumed her law practice.

DVD Illustrations

Chapter 11 DVD

Volume *1* presents edited video clips illustrating the poster session with "Adele's" parents.

Volume *2* presents edited video clips illustrating the poster session with "Brendan" and his mother.

Volume *3* presents edited video clips illustrating poster sessions with "Jack" and his parents.

Chapter 12 *Questions We Are Frequently Asked*

The preceding chapters, the listed references, and the companion DVDs provide the conceptual foundations of the holistic approach to neuropsychological rehabilitation in a "therapeutic community" setting.

Aside from attempting to put together the best clinical program to meet the multiple needs of people with acquired brain injury, we have also attempted to conduct research studies, consistent with our clinical experiences, to provide more scientifically based evidence to support the clinical observations. While the DVDs that accompany different chapters in this volume provide observations, or illustrate key operational and clinical aspects of the program, we published a number of studies that help build part of the scientific scaffold to support the clinical work. (See the list of references.) These publications represent four types of studies: (1) papers concerning the theoretical, or conceptual, underpinnings of holistic neuropsychological rehabilitation, including some publications by others; (2) papers that sought to elucidate the relationships between various (residual) competencies of people with a brain injury and their ability to benefit from remedial and therapeutic interventions; (3) papers about the efficiency of different types of remedial training procedures; and (4) papers related to outcomes, or the effects, of neuropsychological rehabilitative efforts.

In our concluding remarks, we wish to underscore several limitations (or issues) that need to be further clarified by addressing questions we are frequently asked.

1. Which individuals are best suited to the holistic program?

Our program is designed for adults who can participate—in an outpatient setting—in intensive treatment, over extended periods of time, and who have the support of significant others. In our experience, only a relatively small subset of the many traumatically brain-injured individuals possess the cognitive, personality, and interpersonal attributes that make them well suited for this type of holistic program. The issue of whether elements of the program (e.g., its intensity, length, and content) can be disassembled, modified, and applied to individuals who cannot meet these demands remains an open one.

2. Which professionals are best suited to the holistic program?

Only a select number of rehabilitation professionals were found to be best "equipped," in terms of temperament, personality, and versatility of their clinical and didactic skills, to function well in an intense, small-group setting that demands a combination of openness, ability to be part of a team, and the capacity to communicate with patients and their significant others.

3. What resources are necessary to run the program?

The financial resources, the time commitments, as well as the expertise needed to train and supervise a "smoothly" functioning staff are not readily available in many rehabilitation settings. Putting all the pieces into place requires skilled administrative planning and management.

4. How effective has our program been in terms of enabling trainees to resume productive lives?

Studying the outcomes of the first 94 program graduates,[22] it was found that 84% of previously unemployable and unproductive individuals attained the ability to resume productive lives commensurate with their capacity at the time they were discharged from the program. Of these, 63% became competitively employed part-time or full-time, 21% became employed in subsidized capacities, and 16% remained unemployable in any capacity.

5. What constitutes the most effective treatment "package" in a "therapeutic community" program setting?

In a study that was conducted over a period of 2 years,[43] three groups of patients underwent treatments for an identical number of hours (400 hours per 20-week treatment cycle), by the same staff. The three groups received different treatment "mixes" in the same (therapeutic community) setting. The first group received a variety of intensive cognitive remedial training, individualized or in small groups, and personal counseling. The second group received a variety of group "exercises" designed to enhance awareness, self-understanding, and acceptance of limitations imposed by the brain injury, as well as personal counseling. The third group received remedial training to improve cognitive functions, group "exercises" designed to improve awareness and self-understanding, interpersonal communication skills, and personal counseling. While each of the three variations of remedial and therapeutic intervention "packages" has resulted in certain clinically meaningful outcomes, the group that received the most multifocal, or mix, of treatments attained the best outcomes. This treatment "package" was subsequently adopted as the "curriculum" of our program, since it yielded the best overall cognitive personal, vocational, and social adjustments following intensive rehabilitation.

6. Which clinical, demographic, and psychometric factors predict best sought-after outcomes?

A retrospective, multivariate regression analysis[30] revealed that postrehabilitative vocational competence could be predicted by: the duration of unconsciousness; the ability of the patients to self-regulate negative moods and affects, their capacity to empathize with others, the ability to reason abstractly, and their ability to achieve acceptance of the limitations that were imposed by the brain injury. It was further found that nearly half of the approximately 60% of the variance that was accounted for by the combined five "best predictor" variables was contributed by the "acceptance" index alone. While these findings present a useful clinical template for decision making, they are modulated by individual and situational considerations.

7. How important is it to consider the phenomenology (i.e., the subjective experiences) of the person who is undergoing rehabilitation?

In an article published by Diller,[27] he argued that considering the experience of the person who has been receiving rehabilitative treatments is important because it sheds light not only on the question of the extent to which rehabilitative interventions have relieved the person's functional burdens, but also on how the rehabilitant (himself or herself) comes to grips with the limitations that he or she may have to deal with in the future. Considering the rehabilitant's experience can also tell us the personal value, or meaning, that the rehabilitant finds in his or her accomplishments following rehabilitation.

Among his other arguments in favor of considering the "insider's perspective" (i.e., the patient's phenomenology), Diller[27] cites our program's clinical objective, which is in accordance with Goldstein's notion that it is important to help the patient accept limitations voluntarily. Acceptance of limitations is not so much an act of passive "surrender" or defeat, but rather it is the result of an active process of psychological transformation, leading to the recognition by the individual that, despite limitations, one can find meaningful alternatives worth living for.

8. Granted the importance of the subjective experience, is there evidence that objectively measured outcomes of rehabilitation can also be mirrored by the patient's subjective self-appraisal?

A retrospective study of two samples of successful program graduates[8] strongly suggested that a relationship between "external," or objective, measures and "internal," or subjective, self-assessment measures can indeed be shown to exist. It was also hypothesized that self-appraisal ability was related to the Eriksonian construct of ego identity. The relationship between objective and subjective measures of rehabilitation outcomes has recently been confirmed by an international pilot study involving 201 "graduates" of neuropsychological rehabilitation programs from 11 countries.

9. What premorbid personality characteristics could best predict acceptance following a brain injury?

Since our program has been in existence, we have repeatedly observed that program graduates who ultimately achieved acceptance of their limitations, with the greatest degree of equanimity, were those who appeared to share certain common personality characteristics, or traits. Identifying the best candidates who ultimately achieve acceptance through programs providing intensive neuropsychological rehabilitation makes the selection process more rational and efficient.

A study now in progress[44] strongly suggests that program graduates who proved to be the most successful rehabilitants premorbidly

- Were less inclined to experience feelings of angry hostility, depression, self-consciousness, and feelings of vulnerability

- Were more likely to be perceived by others as personally "warm," assertive, as having a positive outlook on life, altruistic, modest, and good (practical) problem solvers

- 10. Preferred going about doing things in an orderly fashion, were self-disciplined, had high achievement needs, and tended to keep their promises

Suggested Readings

1. Barth, J. T., & Boll, T. J. (1981). Rehabilitation and treatment of central nervous system dysfunction: A behavioral medicine perspective. In C. K. Prokop & L. A. Bradley (Eds.), *Medical Psychology*. New York: Academic Press, 242–259.

2. Benton, A. L. (1989). Historical notes on the post concussion syndrome. In H. S. Levin, H. M. Eisenberg, & A. L. Benton (Eds.), *Mild head injury*. New York: Oxford.

3. Ben-Yishay, Y. (1986). Reflections on the evolution of the therapeutic milieu concept. *Neuropsychological Rehabilitation 6*, 327–342.

4. Ben-Yishay, Y. (2000). Post acute neuropsychological rehabilitation. In A. L. Christensen & B. Uzzell (Eds), *International handbook of neuropsychological rehabilitation* (pp. 127–135). New York: Kluwer Academic Plenum.

5. Ben-Yishay, Y. (2007). *Selected early publication on the Holistic Day Program*. New York: N.Y.U. Medical Center, Rusk Institute, BIDTP, BBIRR Publication.

6. Ben-Yishay, Y. (2008). The self and identity in rehabilitation. *Neuropsychological Rehabilitation, 18*(5/6), 513–521.

7. Ben-Yishay, Y., Ben-Nachum, Z., Cohen, A., Gross, Y., Hoofien, D., Rattok, J., et al. (1977). Digest of a two-year comprehensive clinical research program for outpatient head injured israeli veterans. *N.Y.U. Rehabilitation Monograph 64*, 128–176.

8. Ben-Yishay, Y., & Daniels-Zide, E. (2000a). Examined lives: Outcomes after holistic rehabilitation. *Rehabilitation Psychology, 45*(2), 112–129.

9. Ben-Yishay, Y., & Daniels-Zide (2000b). Therapeutic milieu day treatment program. In A. L. Christensen, & B. P. Uzzell (Eds), *International*

handbook of neuropsychological rehabilitation (pp. 183–194). New York: Kluwer/Plenum,.

10. Ben-Yishay, Y., & Diller, L. (1983a). Cognitive deficits. In M. Rosenthal, E. R. Griffith, M. R. Bond, & J. D. Miller (Eds), *Rehabilitation of the head injured adult* (pp. 167–183). Philadelphia: F.A. Davis.

11. Ben-Yishay, Y., & Diller, L. (1983b). Cognitive remediation. In M. Rosenthal, E. R Griffith, M. R. Bond, & J. D. Miller (Eds), *Rehabilitation of the head injured adult* (pp. 367–380). Philadelphia: F.A. Davis.

12. Ben-Yishay, Y., & Diller, L. (1983c). Cognitive remediation in traumatic brain injury: Update and issues. *Archives of Physical Medicine and Rehabilitation 74*, 204–213.

13. Ben-Yishay, Y., & Diller, L. (2008). Kurt Goldstein's holistic ideas–an alternative, or complementary, approach to the management of brain-injured individuals, U.S. *Neurology, 4*(1) 79–80.

14. Ben-Yishay, Y., Diller, L., Gerstman, L., & Gordon, W. (1970). Relationship between initial competence and ability to profit from cues in brain damaged individuals. *Journal of Abnormal Psychology, 75*, 248–259.

15. Ben-Yishay, Y., Diller, L., & Mandleberg, I. (1970). Ability to profit from cues as a function of initial competence in normal and brain-injured adults: A replication of previous findings. *Journal of Abnormal Psychology 76*, 378–379.

16. Ben-Yishay, Y., & Gold, J. (1990). Therapeutic milieu approach to neuropsychological rehabilitation. In R. L. Wood (Ed.), *Neurobehavioral sequelae of traumatic brain injury* (pp. 194–215). London: Taylor and Francis.

17. Ben-Yishay, Y., & Lakin, P. (1989). Structured group treatment for brain injury survivors. In D. W. Ellis & A. L. Christensen (Eds.), *Neuropsychological treatment after brain injury* (pp. 271–295). Boston: Kluwer Academic Publishers.

18. Ben-Yishay, Y., Lakin, P., Ross, B., Rattok, J., Piasetsky, E. B. and Diller, L. (1983). Psychotherapy following severe brain injury: Issues and answers. *N.Y.U. Rehabilitation Monograph, 66*, 128–148.

19. Ben-Yishay, Y., & Prigatano, G. P. (1990). Cognitive remediation. In M. Rosenthal, E. R. Griffith, M. R. Bond, & J. D. Miller (Eds.), *Rehabilitation of the adult and child with traumatic brain injury* (2nd ed., pp. 393–408). Philadelphia: F.A. Davis.

20. Ben-Yishay, Y., Rattok, J., Lakin, P., Piasetsky, E., Ross, B., Silver, S., et al. (1985). Neuropsychological rehabilitation: The quest for a holistic approach. *Seminars in Neurology, 5*, 252–259.

21. Ben-Yishay, Y., Rattok, J., Ross, B., Schaier, A. H., Scherzer, P., & Diller, L. (1979). Structured group techniques for heterogeneous groups of head trauma patients. *N.Y.U. Rehabilitation Monograph*, *60*, 38–88.

22. Ben-Yishay, Y., Silver, S. L., & Piasetsky, E. (1987). Relationship between employability and vocational outcome after intensive holistic cognitive rehabilitation. *Journal of Head Trauma Rehabilitation*. *1*, 35–48.

23. Boll, T. J., O'Leary, D. S., & Barth J.T., (1981). A quantitative and qualitative approach to neuropsychological evaluation. In C. K. Prokop & L. A. Bradley (Eds.), *Medical psychology* (pp. 68–79). New York: Academic Press.

24. Cicerone, K. D., & Wood, J. C. (1987). Planning disorder after closed head injury: A case study. *Archives of Physical Medicine and Rehabilitation*, *68*, 111–115.

25. Diller, L. (1985). Neuropsychological rehabilitation. In M. Meier, A. L. Benton, & L. Diller (Eds.), *Neuropsychological rehabilitation* (pp. 3–17). New York: Guilford.

26. Diller, L. (1994). Finding the right combinations: Changes in rehabilitation over the past five years. In A. L. Christensen, & B. P. Uzzell (Eds.). *brain injury and neuropsychological rehabilitation* (pp. 1–16). Mahwah, NJ: Lawrence Erlbaum.

27. Diller, L. (2004). Pushing the frames of reference in traumatic brain injury rehabilitation. *American Congress of Rehabilitation Medicine*, *86*(6), 1075–1080.

28. Diller, L., & Ben-Yishay, Y. (1988). Stroke and traumatic brain injury: Behavioral and psychosocial considerations. In J. Goodgold (Ed.), *Rehabilitation medicine* (pp. 135–143). Washington, DC: C. V. Mosley.

29. Diller, L., & Gordon, W. (1981). Interventions for cognitive deficits in brain injured adults. *Journal of Consulting and Clinical Psychology 49*, 882–833.

30. Ezrachi, O., Ben-Yishay, Y., & Kay, T. (1991). Predicting employment in traumatic brain injury following neuropsychological rehabilitation. *Journal of Head Trauma Rehabilitation*, *6*(3) 71–84.

31. Goldstein, K. (1942). *After effects of brain injuries in war. Their evaluation and treatment.* New York: Grune and Stratton.

32. Goldstein, K. (1952). *Human nature in the light of psycholopathology.* Cambridge, MA: Harvard University Press.

33. Goldstein K. (1959a). Notes on the development of my concepts. *Journal of Individual Psychology 15*(1), 5–19.

34. Goldstein, K. (1959b). What we can learn from pathology for normal psychology. In G. Leviton (Ed.), *Proceedings of Conference Sponsored by U.S. Dept. of HEW (June 13)*, 36–135.

35. Itard, J. M. G. (1962). *The wild boy of averon* (G. Humphrey, Trans.). New York: Appleton Century Crofts.

36. Levin, H., Benton, A. L., & Grossman, R. G. (1982). *Neurobehavioral consequences of closed head injury.* New York: Oxford University Press.

37. Lezak, M. (1995). *Neuropsychological assessment* (3rd ed.). New York: Oxford University Press.

38. Luria, A. R. (1963). *Restoration of function after brain injury.* New York: Macmillan Co.

39. Luria, A. R. (1966). *Higher cortical functions.* New York: Basic Books.

40. Luria, A. R. (1973). *The working brain.* New York: Basic Books.

41. Prigatano, G. P. (1999). *Principles of neuropsychological rehabilitation.* New York: Oxford University Press.

42. Prigatano, G. P., & Ben-Yishay, Y. (1999). Psychotherapy and psychotherapeutic interventions in brain injury rehabilitation. In M. Rosenthal, E. R. Griffith, J. S. Korntzer, & B. Pentland (Eds.), *Rehabilitation of the adult and child with traumatic brain injury* (3rd ed., pp. 271–283). Philadelphia: F.A. Davis.

43. Rattok, J., Ben-Yishay, Y., & Ezrachi, O. (1992). Outcome of different treatment mixes in a multidimensional neuropsychological rehabilitation program. *Neuropsychology, 6* (4), 395–415.

44. Reyes, A., Margolis, S. A., & Biderman, D. J. (2009). *Premorbid predictors of successful rehabilitation outcomes following traumatic brain injury.* Publication pending.

45. Ross, B., Ben-Yishay, Y., Lakin, P., Rattok, J., Thomas, J. L., & Diller, L. (1982). Using a "therapeutic community" to modify the behavior of head trauma patients. *N.Y.U. Rehabilitation Monograph, 64,* 181–195.

46. Sohlberg, M. M., & Mateer, C. A. (1989). *Introduction to cognitive rehabilitation.* New York: Guilford.

47. Stein, D. G., Brailowski, S., & Will, B. (1995). *Brain repair.* New York: Oxford University Press.

Index

Note: Page references followed by "*f*" and "*t*" denote figures and tables, respectively.